IF NATUROPATHS ARE "QUACKS"... THEN I GUESS I'M A DUCK

Confessions of a Naturopath

by

SHAUNA K. YOUNG, PHD, CTN

Original Release: 2008
Revised: 2012

ISBN: 1470093359
ISBN 13: 9781470093358

Library of Congress Control Number: 2012903244
CreateSpace, North Charleston, SC

For you Dad.
We built it, and they come.
A lot of them…

About the Author

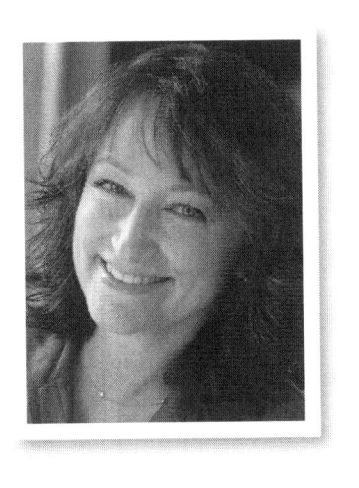

Shauna K. Young,
Ph.D., CTN, CBS, OSJ

Shauna Young is the owner and Medical Director of the Assertive Wellness Research Center in Durango, CO, which first opened its doors in 2001. Since its humble beginnings, her Center has now to date had the unique pleasure of seeing many thousands of clients who have had the confidence to travel from every U.S. State and even several foreign countries based almost exclusively on referrals from other practitioners and from clients who have been pleased with the consultation, products and help.

Shauna completed her initial education and obtained her degree as a Naturopath under a regimented correspondence curriculum through the Herbal Healer Academy, a school certified by the American Naturopathic Medical Association (ANMA). Since 2001, she has been practicing as a Traditional Naturopath within the disciplines of her continuing education and certification with the American Naturopathic Certification Board and as a Certified Biofeedback Specialist (CBS) with the Natural Therapies Certification Board.

In 2005, after four years of clinical observations and experience, Shauna began specific research regarding her theorized negative effects of excess and stored manganese on the human neurological and sensory input systems and its possible symptomatic connections to Autism and other neurological, learning and behavioral disorders in both children and adults. The unique success of this clinical research, originally referred to as "The Popeye Protocol" and currently as the "Spectrum Balance® Protocol", led to her receiving numerous speaking engagements and accolades including two Distinguished Awards of Excellence from the internationally recognized Global Foundation for Integrative Medicine.

Shauna holds a Bachelor of Science Degree in Natural Sciences and based on the merits of her research, theories and doctoral thesis on manganism as it relates to Autism, was earned a Doctor of Philosophy (PhD) in Natural Sciences from the University of Natural Medicine in Santa Fe, New Mexico. In February of 2008 she was also knighted into the international Sovereign Medical Order of the Knights Hospitaller in recognition of the unique impact of her work with Autism and for positively advancing the field of natural medicine in general. The mission of the Knights Hospitaller is to promote higher levels of international health and to establish, equip, staff and maintain humanitarian and medical treatment centers worldwide.

She has also been appointed to the faculty of the University of Natural Medicine in Santa Fe, NM and serves as the Chief Medical Advisor for the NoHarm Foundation (www.noharm-foundation.org), a Colorado not-for-profit organization formed with the primary goal of disseminating the highly important information resulting from Dr. Young's work with the intent of ushering in a new paradigm in research and providing real help for countless children and adults suffering with Autism disorders. This is expected to serve as a lighting rod issue to create permanent positive change in how the role and importance of natural medicine is perceived by the public and peer medical communities.

Shauna also maintains membership with the American Association of Nutritional Consultants, is an Advisory Board Member for the Colorado Chapter of the Coalition for Natural Health, and is a member and serves as Chairperson of the Legislative & Legal Fund of the Colorado Naturopathic Medical

Association. For a number of years now she has been an international lecturer on many aspects of natural medicine, health freedom issues, the Spectrum Balance® Protocol, Autism Spectrum Disorders and many other health related topics. "*If Naturopaths Are Quacks, Then I Guess I'm a Duck*", is Shauna Young's first authored book, and she is currently working on her second that will specifically focus on and chronicle her research and uniquely successful work with Autism Spectrum Disorders.

Disclosure & Disclaimer Statement

This book is offered for informational, educational and entertainment purposes only. As Dr. Shauna Young is not a medical doctor (M.D.), she does not give out what is legally referred to as "medical advice". If you have any known medical conditions, please consult with your doctor before making any significant changes in your diet, supplementation, medications, exercise or other lifestyle aspects.

Understand that sources of health-related information other than that supplied by paid actors in TV commercials advertising prescription drugs, may be dangerous to your health, or at least to the health of the pharmaceutical industry. Therefore, proceed at your own risk.

As your ability to positively influence your own health and that of your family represents dangerous competition to the medical establishment and levels of personal empowerment that many people are uncomfortable with, be aware that any attempts you make to proactively improve your health will be met with re-sistance and ridicule from certain medical practitioners, in-laws, hairdressers and co-workers. Just be aware that <u>all</u> of them are more intelligent than you are and know more about your own body than you do.

Rest assured that your friendly government will always know best regarding your personal health needs and choices, and un-derstands far more about the needs of your children than you do as merely their parents. Just who do you think you are anyway?

Be forewarned that if one more person asks us if person-al decisions such as to cook with more olive oil than soybean oil or to eat more sweet potatoes than white potatoes are "FDA Approved", Dr. Young is liable to smack them up side the head.

Don't taunt Dr. Young.

Please don't take anything Dr. Young says as gospel. Extend the same caution to all other sources for such vitally important information. Always do your own research, put on your big-boy or big-girl pants, and then reach your own conclusions and decisions. If you neglect or refuse to exercise such freedom and control over your own life, then we have a long and growing list of corporations and government agencies that will be very happy to do it for you.

Thank you

Order of Contents

"Naturopathy": One Definition

A distinct system of non-invasive healthcare and health assessment in which neither surgery nor drugs are used; dependence being placed instead on education, counseling, naturopathic modalities and natural substances, including without limitation, the use of foods, food extracts, vitamins, minerals, enzymes, digestive aids, botanical substances, topical natural substances, homeopathic preparations, air, water, heat, cold, sound, light, the physical modalities of magnetic therapy, naturopathic non-manipulative bodywork and exercise to help stimulate and maintain the individual's intrinsic self-healing processes.

"The natural force within each of us is that greatest healer of all."

— HIPPOCRATES

CHAPTER 1

Who Am I?

"The necessity of teaching mankind not to take drugs and medicines is a duty incumbent upon all who know their uncertainty and injurious effects; and the time is not far distant when the drug system will be abandoned."

— CHARLES ARMBRUSTER, M.D.

NAME: Shauna Young

BORN: Orange County, California

TURN-ONS: Moonlight walks on the beach, cuddly dogs, green-eyed men, and people who change their diets when I ask them to without too much whining.

TURN-OFFS: Cat boxes, Brussels sprouts and the answer, "I don't know" when I ask someone why he or she has had an organ removed.

But seriously folks...
Who am I, *really*?

Well, when I received my initial certification and credential in 2001, I was an N.D., a Naturopathic Doctor. This week for some mysterious reason, I'm now a C.T.N., a Certified Traditional Naturopath. Next week I may be something else; who knows. The name and label may change, but the work doesn't. Therefore it doesn't really matter to me. It just gets to be a tad expensive printing new business cards every time some government agency changes their mind or one of our naturopathic associations caves in (yet again) to try to "avoid problems." But then again, Echinacea by any other name will still clean your blood, so...

The "powers that be" are constantly trying to make it very clear to people that we Naturopaths aren't "real doctors," *i.e.* MD's, which is fine with me. I have no desire to be an MD. I don't want to do what they do, and I'm certainly not trained for it. As for the "real doctor" part, since a doctor is defined as a "teacher" or "practitioner in the healing arts" it seems to me that I *am* a real doctor, whatever "they" decide to call me. I, Shauna Young, am a doctor of natural medicine. But as I said, as long as people know I'm here to be a healer, I really don't care what moniker they use.

Although, since "they" (as most seem to call them) keep making it so difficult for Naturopaths to continue to practice, I also attained a Doctor of Philosophy (PhD) in Natural Sciences, so I'm actually *two* doctors! So there...

When I first became a Naturopath, I somehow assumed that I'd be working with people who were healthy for the most part, and who just wanted some advice on diet, exercise, lifestyle and what supplements they should take. That happy little thought flew out the window during only my second month in practice.

One day, I came face to face with a sweet little woman who was in a wheelchair and was catheterized. She was in Stage 4 ovarian cancer. Her doctor had given her between three and six weeks to live and wanted to put her on morphine. Since the idea of being in a drug-induced delirium for the remainder of her life didn't much appeal to her, she asked if I had something else she might do. After telling her I didn't have a whole lot in the way of straight painkillers, I did what naturopaths do; I did what I could to get her natural immune system to reactivate. Apparently it did, and after she was able to get out of her wheelchair three months later and walk into her church, I suddenly found myself with quite a clientele of very sick people.

So mostly who I continue to see from that point forward are *not* the healthy people seeking basic advice that I first imagined, but rather a sometimes seemingly endless line of desperately ill and many times psychologically hopeless people. Walkers and wheelchairs and oxygen tanks – oh my! People who have been thrown away by western medicine – often told to "Go home and get their affairs in order", or that they will "never recover", or that no one simply has any idea what's wrong with them. I wasn't exactly sure why I was getting so many of these people until my brother/business manager handed me the answer one day. "Why am I getting all these incredibly sick people who want me to fix them?" I whined on one exceedingly busy day. "Because you *can*" he answered. And it's true.

We are effective here. We work on simple and effective principles. Stimulate and balance the immune system, get toxicity and other obstacles to healing out of the way, and try to let the body take care of itself. Also, I *care* about my clients and they know it, and I don't spook easily. If a person has made the decision to fight his or her disease or condition, then I get on the team and do my best to fight right along with him or her. Sometimes people just need a coach and/or teammate.

The reason I wrote this book is twofold: First and foremost is because I want you to know that you and only you are the final arbiter of your health. Your doctors (including me) are there to give advice, but YOU make the final decision. So make it a good one. Consider all your options, and then make the call that you believe in and that makes you comfortable and get on with it. And second: I really want you to know what Naturopaths do, and that we're even out there. I was once asked by a 38-year-old hairdresser what I did for a living. I replied, "I'm a Naturopath." She had absolutely no idea what this meant, and when I explained it to her, she was aghast. "You mean people do that for a living?" Yes we do. And in <u>most</u> States, we're right there in the phone book under "Naturopaths." Check yours.

So putting aside all the titles, names and degrees for a moment, who am I *really*?

Some people say I'm far too serious, while others assert that I'm actually a loony. I guess I can find it within myself to agree with both sides of that issue, depending on which day you ask me. You'll probably notice in the course of this book that I go a long way to avoid talking too much about my own personal history, personal beliefs or political leanings and I'll tell you why. I don't want you to view this book as a story about me, Shauna Young. I want you to read this book as the story of a Naturopath – of a person who works in a field that you may not know much about, every day. My personal story, the color of my hair, what I formerly did with my time or even how I got here are not the message I'm trying to convey. Not the "me" that I want you to get to know.

Instead, I want you to know the person with this mission: I want you to know that there are always *choices* available to you for your healthcare. This is my true story – no one else's. And although my sense of humor is questionable and has even been called "dark" at times, it's what has kept me going through the quagmire of health catastrophes I've witnessed and the constantly changing minefield of legal regulations we navigate through, so please indulge me if I try to tell this story with as much humor as I can. I'm telling it to you this way because I want to make you laugh, and maybe make you cry, but mostly I just want you to know that YOU DO HAVE CHOICES.

There are alternatives to the "cut, poison and burn" mentality that is so prevalent in allopathic medicine, and I hope that this book will encourage you to seek out and consider all your options. Investigate them thoroughly and then see what you think. And speaking of investigation, you're going to see a lot of places where I give some info, and than advise you to "look it up yourself." I am being literal about this. Please, question what I am saying – be my guest. Go to the PDR (Physicians' Desk Reference) either by looking at the book available from any pharmacist (if you can lift it), or go online. Use a search engine, or visit a website such as www.rxlist.com and *look it all up*. Knowledge is power. Get some.

Like all non-empirical evidence, this book is anecdotal. All I really know is that an awful lot of people have walked in here sick, and then have walked out well. If that's an *anecdote* then I'll take it. It's an anecdote for a healer to be proud of.

CHAPTER 2

Doing it My Way

""The definition of insanity is doing the same thing over and over and expecting different results."

— BENJAMIN FRANKLIN

Before I delve into the case studies and statistics, I think it's important that you get an idea of how I work. It's a little different than a lot of folks (even other Naturopaths) and my team and I have found it to be the synergistic basis of our success, and more important, the health success of our clients.

The Surroundings

First of all, contrary to what many envision as the stereotypical atmosphere of a natural practitioner, my office looks like, well, an office. Chairs, magazines, prints of flowers or other paintings on the walls, radio playing in the background. Please understand that I'm *not* dissing those who choose to decorate their office with chakra charts, beads, posters of various deities, and play sitar music. In fact, that can all be rather relaxing and nice. It's just that we decided to *market* our services to a different demographic, and it's difficult to attract them when you have an atmosphere that makes so many people feel out of their element and comfort level.

Specifically, I and my healthcare team made a conscious decision to create a place for the type of folks who may have never in their lives considered going outside the accepted "norm," and this group is often made a little uneasy in the presence of, what one of my clients calls, "all that New Age-y stuff." Besides, my spiritual/political or any other "...als" or "...isms" really aren't anyone else's business or concern, so why wear them in my office? I find that most of my clients are sufficiently weirded-out just by being *in the office* of an "alternative practitioner", so we do our best to make them feel as surrounded by their familiar comfort zone as possible.

Of course this runs the risk of somewhat cutting me off from the people who *do* feel more comfortable with the iconic trappings of New Age decor, but I feel that these folks have plenty of choices out there, and you can't have it both ways. Besides, my personal style is a little more "in your face", which likely doesn't quite mesh with soothing flute music.

The Consultation Process

My first session with someone is a full hour long and usually includes a test procedure with a piece of bio-resonant equipment. I always spend an hour with the first visit, and a minimum of a half hour on follow-up visits. This may seem like a lot of time to some (and "the land where time stands still" to medical doctors), but I feel that it takes time to hear what people are really trying to say. Although you've probably heard of the "third eye," I often feel that I am listening with my "third ear" – not just to the words and symptoms, but to the overall feeling of who this person really is. This gives me a very good idea of what kind of shape his or her body might be in, and what we will have to work on in the foreseeable future.

From this point (for about 99% of clients) we start with organ/filter detoxification. It's amazing how little attention most people pay to their own body filters: Liver, kidneys, bowel and lymph. Look at it this way; you wouldn't think of getting the oil changed in your car without changing the filters – that would be silly! After all, if you put clean oil on top of a dirty filter, you get...dirty oil. A big waste of time and money. So likewise, throwing perfectly good (and sometimes expensive) supplements in on top of dirty body filters can amount to the same thing.

Assessing the Client Type

With any client/patient-related service that you've been at for a while, and I've been at this more than ten years, you recognize (often in the first consultation) certain types of people. Some types need more work and attention than others, and this has nothing to do for my purposes with their health status per se. It's more *who* they are. But working with them successfully is what I signed on to do, even if I want to vent my occasional frustration on a punching bag. Below I describe several very different categories of people, not in any way to poke fun at them, but to show how a little applied observation can better help me to help them. Hopefully you'll find these profiles both amusing and educational.

The Self-Medicators: These folks can be a real problem; not to me as much as to themselves. One of the reasons why many people think that natural supplements don't work is because they are self-medicators, and in many cases, self-*over*-medicators. The supplements they tried "didn't work" because of a large variety of reasons. I'll just hit the top few.

First; as I mentioned, if your filters are clogged up, chances are the supplements never really made their way into your system in the first place. They never had a fair shot. They went straight to the body elimination phase without ever passing "Go" (although they may have collected $200 or so).

Second; due to the inordinate amount of hype that surrounds the sales and use of supplements, many people are dissatisfied with the "real world" outcome they achieved which greatly pales in comparison to the often extravagant claims made on a label or website. Looking at the claims that manufacturers often make for many supplements will boggle the senses (especially the common sense). Even though someone might actually feel somewhat better (maybe something as subtle as just having more overall energy), many feel disappointed that after an entire month on their "Wonder-Vites" or "Mega-Ultra-Aminos" that they *still* don't have the stamina to run a marathon. By the way, I love hearing that phrase, "I still don't..." after only a *month*. Pretty short "still" period if you ask me, as they have many times developed their health problems over years and even decades.

Third; mostly due to this hype (and to the desperation many feel that there has to be *something* out there that will help) about 85% of supplements are being used inappropriately and/or for conditions for which they are not known to be effective in the first place. It's amazing how often when I ask why someone is taking a particular supplement, he or she responds, "It's supposed to be good for you." Good for what exactly? If you're not sure, then how do you know whether it's been effective or not?

Fourth; and this happens often, self-medicators just aren't taking good quality supplements in the first place. This leads to yet another reason to seek guidance with your health because not all natural products are created equally. Because vitamins and supplements are such big moneymakers nowadays, numerous companies (including pharmaceutical companies that perhaps prefer that they *don't* work to any great degrees) have jumped onto the lucrative supplement bandwagon. That bottle of melatonin you got with the "Nature's Basket of Bunnies" label on it could just as easily be a cheap Big Pharma product, as it could be from a *real* nutritional supplement company.

And unfortunately a lot of these are shoddily made supplements are either without sufficient amounts of ingredients to make them work, or with so many additives and fillers that nullify any good they could possibly do. The only upside of these products is that they tend to be *cheap*, so a lot of people try them first to "see if they work." They don't. The products that my practice and most Naturopathic practices work with are all well-researched and effective products, and many of them are only available through healthcare professionals. That way their makers know someone actually has their eye on you, and knows what they're used for!

An analogy I often give to clients, especially to self-medicators, is that of a farmer. If you want a crop to grow, you don't just walk outside, fling a handful of seeds on the ground and expect a crop to propagate. Only a bonehead would expect that strategy to work. Instead you prepare the field. You till, water and fertilize first, then you plant seeds, water some more, and then watch it grow. In a human being this process can take some time, and more than one client tired of cleansing has groaned to me, "Am I ready to be planted yet?"

The List Makers: In general, I like lists. A list helps a person organize his or her thoughts, be clear and remember important things in a session. In fact, I'm a big list maker myself. However, I'm not talking about these short, helpful and to-the-point lists. I'm speaking about the *Dreaded Lists from Hell* that let you know that these people have very little else of priority in their lives than sitting around and unfortunately obsessing on every minute detail of themselves and their health.

If you are a health care provider of any kind, I'm sure the hair just went up on the back of your neck at my mention of List Makers. We've all seen them and know them for the wake-up-and-smell-the-obsession call to action that they are. When you encounter a List Maker you know you're in trouble, and if that unholy list is...heaven forbid...*typed*...gulp! In my experience, these people are nearly impossible to satisfy on any level, because no matter how many items you're able to blast off their list, there are always more. Their migraines, digestive issues and joint pain may have disappeared, but they still have that "ear that gets sore when I sleep on my side" to keep you humble! Please keep in mind; these are not symptoms like "I often have a headache in the morning," or "Citrus foods seem to make my stomach hurt." Really, I actually like and appreciate those kinds of lists! No, the stuff I'm talking about is more along the lines of:

"The cuticle on the inside of my left thumb is nearly always dry."
"Sometimes I get a tiny dry spot on my scalp under my hair."
"My stomach sometimes feels funny."

"I feel tired in the morning if I stay up too late."

"I sometimes get a sour stomach from a certain brand of carrots."

"My eyelashes seem dry."

"My left nostril hurts sometimes for a second or so when I blow my nose."

These are all real – I pulled them straight from client charts.

The "I Feel Funny" Folks: Sure, I understand that trying to convey to a doctor that something isn't quite right is sometimes difficult. However, the "feels funny" thing is nearly always a bad sign when I hear it. I say, "Does it hurt?" They ponder for a moment. "No... not really *pain...*" I try again. "Irritation? Nerve sensation? Fullness? Tickling? Pressure...?" Again the careful thought. "No... not really any of those, it's just a *funny* feeling". Great – I'll get right on that.

The "sometimes", "not really", or "rarely" are bad markers as well. If someone can recall something that happens for a fleeting moment once in a blue moon well enough to put it in a typed list, then chances are he or she is going to be dang near impossible to satisfy. Again – being *realistic* is very important.

And speaking of being realistic – You can't imagine how many people have come into my office with long, *long* standing medical conditions (like the fifty five year old woman who recently told me that she had been sick since 8th grade), an "incurable" disease, or in 4th Stage cancer, who are absolutely incensed that:

A. They are expected to pay me for my advice and supplements
B. That I won't give them an *exact date* when they will feel well
C. That I won't "guarantee" that they will get well at all
D. That I ask them to make dietary and lifestyle changes

It would blow your mind to know how often this type of person has appeared in my office! As crazy as it sounds, they aren't even rare. Such people, who generally have seen multiple health care providers (sometimes a dozen or more), have "tried everything" to get well, and have spent up to decades of being ill, are generally the first ones to complain about cost, and to use the dreaded "still" word.

As in…

Me: "So how are you doing"?

Them: "I'm *still* tired and achy".

Me: "Well you've had Lyme Disease for 12 years…"

Them: "Yeah, but I just still don't feel good. How long is this going to take"?

Me: "More than 30 days".

Them: Embarrassed silence…sometimes…if I'm lucky…

The "Yes, buts": Everything you say to a "Yes, but" person, whether it's about food, water consumption, exercise programs, ways to get better sleep or have more energy is followed by, "Yes, but…" This is both non-productive and annoying, and frankly, I don't get it. Why come in, have an appointment, ask and pay me for my opinion, then immediately counter every word that comes out of my mouth? Sorry to be sexist, but it's usually a man, and it usually goes something like this:

Them: "I get these stomach aches after lunch almost every day."

Me: "What do you usually have for lunch?"

Them: (hesitantly) "Well, there's a (insert name of a fast food chain here) right next to my office, so I usually grab a burger or something."

Me: "Well, I'm sure I don't have to tell you that fast food isn't the best for your…"

Them: (cutting me off) "*Yes, but* I only get 20 minutes for lunch, so that's all I have time for."

Me: "So not only are you eating a greasy burger and fries, you're wolfing it down in less than 20 minutes? That's not really…"

THEM: "*Yes, but* that's all the time I get. If I take longer I could get fired."

ME: "Okay, then maybe we should figure out how you can pack a lunch from home that will be less..."

THEM: (cutting me off...again) "*Yes, but* then I'd have to get up earlier to make lunch, and I'm already tired from having a stomach ache all night..."

And on, and on, and *on*. After about twenty minutes of this from one guy, I leaned back in my chair and said, "Tell you what. You tell me what you ARE willing to do, and I'll see if I can help you at all based upon that because you obviously aren't interested in my input." At first he looked puzzled, then embarrassed. He did however let me tell him what I thought he needed to do for nearly a minute and a half without any "Yes, buts..." so I guess I got my point across. Well, as much as he let me.

If a client is any one of these types, I just work my best to understand him or her and then adapt how I further explain my protocols and the results they realistically should expect – "realistic" being a really big factor.

Dietary Rules (and How I Became a Cavewoman)

For many years, a staple of my work was the Blood Type Diet (the original 1996 work by Peter D'Adamo). This is not really a "diet" in the way that people usually think of the term; that is, it's not just for *weight loss*. Rather, the concept of the Blood Type Diet is more about putting gasoline into the tank of a vehicle with a gasoline engine, instead of diesel fuel. Both fuel types can be effective, but only when the right type of fuel is used to power the respective engine. I also have a tendency to prefer the "lifestyle change" type of dietary strategies over weight loss-type diets, so the blood type science appealed to me on that level as well.

However, over the years I have come to find the Blood Type Diet more and more... shall we say, *iffy*. I loved the foundational research and data put into the first book, but the last one?

Instead of information on lectins and food sugars, it was focusing more on measuring your finger lengths and breaking you down into groups like "The Nomad", "The Warrior" or "The Teacher". As my brother Doug asked, "Where are 'The Couch Potato' and 'The Pole Dancer' types?" I think it's tough to preserve one's credibility while measuring someone's fingers...

Having said that, I do want to be clear that I still think that there's a lot of merit to the Blood Type Diet. I was a vegetarian (for six endless, depressing months) before starting the Type O Diet in 1996 and did very well on it for a long time. For one thing, figuring out that my body ran much more effectively by giving it red meat was quite a blessing! This was the best science out there at the time, and I have thousands of clients who significantly changed and improved their lives using it.

One thing I continued to observe throughout the years was concerns and issues with grains. Being an O blood type, I was allowed certain grains like rice, Ezekiel bread, etc. in my diet, but over the years I found myself cutting them more and more from my life. Especially as I left my forties and drifted into my fifties I noticed that grains of any type were not only a struggle for my figure, but for my fatigue. Even now, eleven years into practice, my schedule is as grueling (or more so) as it ever was, and I started finding myself a little low on energy. It also became clear to me over the years that by far I wasn't the only one feeling that way. A common occurrence is for clients who were strictly adhering to the Blood Type Diet to continue to struggle with their weight; especially that pesky last 10 pounds. Perplexing...

Five years into practice, as I started to write my own diet primarily intended for children with Autism Spectrum and related disorders (more about that in Chapter 12) I found that I had a lot more compassion for Peter D'Adamo! Here I was trying to create a dietary protocol that is *healing the body and mind*, and I have all these people giving me frustrating input like "You *have* to include bread! What about hot dogs? My child will die without macaroni and cheese"! Although I suspected that including any kind of pasta, rice or even cheese might slow down the process, I eventually bent to include minor portions within the diet or most people would never have agreed to even start it in the first place! D'Adamo probably had his "perfect diet" in mind too, but had to include some "*iffy*" things just to get people to try it. So prop's to D'Adamo...

As for the ongoing evolution of my own dietary plan, a funny thing was happening. Understand that as of the current date this diet has been downloaded over the Internet and used by thousands of people in more than 60 countries, so obviously I've never even met the vast majority of families that I help and work with by phone, email and even anonymously, and therefore have had little idea about things occurring in each family other than with the particular child in question. Since I have always encouraged the entire family to be on the same diet for the good of their affected child, I would hear the occasional "I like this diet too" or "My husband has lost 20 pounds" or something random like that, but during appointments I'm generally only focused on and discussing the ASD-affected child or adult.

Then we received a particular email from a parent. Apparently this guy had been on our Spectrum Balance® Protocol Diet along with his Autistic son for about four months when he went in to get a regular medical check up. The so-called "hereditary" LDL cholesterol issues that his doctors had told him he would always have, had dropped by 137 points. "Is this common?" he asked me.

Huh...I really wasn't sure! So I started pulling some client charts and calling parents to ask about their broader experiences with the diet. "Oh..." they told me, "I've lost thirty five pounds" or "My arthritis went away", "My asthma went away", "My PMS went away", "My eczema I've had since high school went away" and on and on, and on. Gosh folks, you think you might have mentioned that to me? It certainly would have been helpful in my research! Oh well...

So here I have a diet where I tell you to eat more meat, eggs and healthy fats, and people have weight, cholesterol, blood pressure, blood sugar and allergy issues falling off them like ducks shedding water. Sounds counterintuitive doesn't it? And yet, facts is facts. Yes, it's an anti-inflammatory diet, but still it seemed like an awful lot of good coming from just that aspect alone. Again I was wishing for labs and white coats and research dollars to investigate it more fully, but alas, no money for the Naturopath. I had to be contented with the fact that it *does* work without me necessarily understanding it completely.

In my sixth year of using my own diet (patience, patience, Chapter 12…), my sister-in-law, Lori, who is also the weight loss counselor at our center, handed me a book saying "This guy explains why your diet is working so well". "This guy" as it turns out, was Robb Wolf, and he certainly did help explain my diet perfectly in his book "The Paleo Solution". As it turns out, I had developed and was advising a predominantly "Paleo" dietary philosophy and didn't even know it.

Since Robb's book and others on the subject explain it so logically and beautifully, I won't attempt to go into this newly evolving science fully in this book, but I will explain the important basics from my perspective. Paleo is short for "Paleolithic" and represents the blossoming and derivative dietary philosophies that have primarily resulted from the initial theories and work of Loren Cordain, PhD. There is excellent and building evidence that mankind's transitions away from Paleo "Caveman-type" diets, initially beginning with the current Neolithic period considered to by around 10,000 years ago, have not only led to largely different food mix and sources of "modern" nutrition, but have greatly contributed to much of the malnutrition and disease that we see today. It seems that our human bodies just may neither have been designed nor have even yet adequately adapted to eat diets that more modern cultures have found through agriculture to be most manageable, economical and convenient.

Following Paleo practices, you eat meats of all types, vegetables, fruit, good fats and nuts. No grains, no legumes and limited or no dairy (based on sensitivity). Portion size and even calorie counting is far less important than the simple exclusion of the problematic foods. I like the fact that even though you'll find many references to Paleo "diet(s)", this truly represents a *lifestyle* eating philosophy that is in no way suggested as some short-term fix for weight issues alone that you'll soon discard and want to return to your old eating habits.

The more I investigated this way of eating, the more I liked it. And the more you seriously look into dietary science and the "whole grains and fiber thing", the further down the rabbit hole you go. As it turns out, a massive amount of the research and "studies" that have been done on the health benefits of grains are not independent studies, but rather trials that are sponsored and funded by the same companies that produce and market grain products. This has started me on a whole other course of education/ranting: How to distinguish an actual "health food" from an advertising campaign! Like I needed something else to do.

Anything new introduced into my practice usually follows the same procedure, and the Paleo type diet was no exception: I try it on myself first, then our staff, then clients. In my own case I doubted if I would notice anything significant, since grains in my diet were already minimal. The occasional rice (usually with Sushi), rice pasta, a tortilla here and there, not much really.

Boy was I wrong!

Before I start this recap, a word needs to be said here about my physical condition so you can better understand my experience. At 5'5" I started this process as a size 2. Not as much energy as I wanted, and not as toned as I'd like to be (hey! I sit in a chair all day!), but still a size 2. Not bad...

Week 1: At first I felt really hungry. As I have a pretty big appetite anyway, this is saying something! So I just kept eating... and eating, but only the right foods. So what happened to my weight with all this extra eating? I lost 2 pounds.

Week 2: My appetite returned to normal for the most part and I was finding it very easy to stick to the meat/veggie/fruit/nut thing. Since everyone in our office and a significant number of other volunteers were all on the program, it was actually kind of fun. I started making recipes out of Sarah Fragoso's great cookbook "Everyday Paleo" and was definitely finding my way rapidly.

Week 3: Although only down a few pounds, people started asking me if I'd been working out a lot. And what was that on my stomach? Was that… muscle? Maybe not a six-pack, but definitely the beginning of something! I tried to show this to my staff, but I think it was a little TMI for them. My weight stayed pretty much the same, but my muscle structure was becoming much more clearly defined. Interesting…

Week 4: Yep, definitely muscle was showing. The most significant difference now however, was that I actually felt like getting some exercise. With all the hours I put in with work, writing, traveling, it is very easy to say to yourself "No wonder I'm tired". But suddenly, I actually felt like doing something after work. Amazing…

About two months into eating strictly Paleo, I did something I haven't done in five years. I went on vacation. Yep, left the office, went on vacation and had to eat out every night. And you know what? I didn't gain an ounce. When was the last time that happened to <u>you</u>? SCORE……!!

Oh, and my clothes? Size 0; and not a skinny size 0. Looking pretty fit for an old gal if I do say so myself. Didn't lose much weight (thank goodness), but I lost all the lumps (any woman over forty knows what I'm talking about). My Mom told me she got my Christmas clothes from Barbie's Malibu Condo…

The best part for me though isn't the way I look, but rather the way I feel. Clear head (thinking), clear head (sinus), perfect digestion, boundless energy. Who could ask for more?

So yes, I was a solid Blood Type advocate and now I'm teaching Spectrum Balance® and/or strictly Paleo – An evolution of sorts; or maybe a *de-evolution*? I'm now recommending our adaptations of Paleo diets to all my clients to some mixed comments. Most of them are loving it as much as I am, but a few die hards really want to hold on to the few breads and pastas that the Blood Type Diet allows. I had someone actually yelling at me the other day about it. "You've always been Blood Type and now you're Paleo all of a sudden? You can't do that"!

Yes I can. And I did. As an effective health care provider I feel it absolutely required to always keep an open mind and to always be looking for the better mouse trap so to speak. There is constantly new and better information coming out and I always try my best to stay on top of it. Lest we forget, "everyone" used to think that the world was flat. Enough said...

My Simple Weight Loss Philosophy

Most popular weight loss diets today are based upon calorie counting, portion control, low glycemic indexes, carb restrictions and the like. From my clinical observations, a flaw around these diets is the common misconception and acceptance that if a food is *low-cal*, it's fine and superior to eat. I even see many of these diets suggesting the use of artificial sweeteners because they have no calories! Artificial sweeteners will be discussed (at length) later in this book, but let me just say here that one of the charming aspects of these poisons is that they keep you dehydrated, and I'm here to tell you that dehydration is one of the main reasons that many people have trouble losing weight in the first place. It also needs to be noted that most low-fat or non-fat foods do more harm than good. If you're eating nothing but non-fat foods you're going to wind up deficient in essential fatty acids, thereby setting the stage for increased inflammation in your body. However, that's another can of fish oils...

I'm often told, "Oh, we don't have to worry about my diet. I only eat organic food." Well, that's great, but the *quality* of the food is only part of it. It also needs to be the *right food*. If you take even the finest-grade, most expensive olive oil in the world and poured it into the gas tank of your car, it would still kill your car. Great quality, wrong fuel.

All I know, is that the *only* way that I've ever gotten anyone to lose weight that actually stayed off, is by changing their *lifestyle*. Unless someone is honestly willing to do that, all they're doing is repeating the same mistakes over and over with the same predictable and disappointing results.

As for the quality of your food, that one's easy. The more you spend on organic groceries, the less you spend at the doctor. End of story. Hippocrates said it first and best: "Let food be your medicine." And it's still true.

Cooking at Home

After discussing dietary philosophy and strategy, I talk to clients about how to cook and prepare food. I got a funny email once that said, "God created salad, so the devil created Ranch dressing." Funny, but true.

Easily stated; sautéed, steamed or baked is always better than fried, olive oil and coconut oil are better than butter – although butter is far better than margarine. You can even locate "grass fed" butter now, which is really what you want, so just check the labels. Margarine, in case you haven't seen the research, is way too close molecularly to Tupperware® for me to suggest that anyone actually eat it. That's why it doesn't melt in a microwave.

Speaking of those rotten things, don't get me started on microwave ovens. Yes, they're fast and thus save so much time, but frankly, I'd rather wait for a 40 watt bulb Easy-Bake Oven to do the trick before I'd use one of these contraptions. Lest anyone forget, a microwave oven cooks using *radiation*. They should be called "Radiation Ovens", but I'll bet that would put a real dent in sales! In a fairly well publicized case in Oklahoma (1991 lawsuit regarding one Norma Levitt), a patient died as a result of the use of a microwave for a mere few seconds to heat up blood used for her transfusion. Ten seconds in a microwave was enough to turn blood to poison!

In independent studies in both Switzerland and Russia, researchers found that cooking in a microwave changes the molecular structure enough to turn virtually any healthy foods (and even water) into indigestible and/or unrecognizable carcinogens. If you want to look this up, the Swiss studies (Dr. Blanc and Dr. Hertel) were conducted at the Swiss Federal Institute of Biochemistry and the University Institute for Biochemistry, and the Russian investigations were published by the Atlantis Rising Educational Center, Portland, OR.

But, wait! There's more! Microwave ovens have also been found to depolarize and demagnetize brain tissue (causing lack of focus and memory loss), decrease white blood cell production (decreasing immune response), and alter or over time shut down both male and female hormone production levels (so long libido and hello PMS among other things). And you were worried about living near power lines!

Strong statements? You betcha! If this seems far-fetched or out of line to you, then I encourage you to locate and read all the studies for yourself.

The Taste Issue

Often in this point of discussion, diet, foods and supplements, a client who has years of poor dietary practices (think junk and fast food galore), will give me a hangdog look and weight-of-the-world sigh, then ask: "But, Shauna, does any of this stuff actually *taste* good?"

A good thing to quickly get over and discard is the way-wrong adage that if something is good for you, it has to taste bad. When I start to talk to people about food and supplements, I still get the old, "I know, if it tastes good spit it out." This is both silly and self-defeatist. A few of the extracts and supplements I give people don't taste like champagne, but why should they? After all, they aren't meant for sticking an umbrella in and drinking at a cocktail party, they're for ingesting and creating a positive response in your body. So get over it. Don't worry so much about the taste and just be happy for how you feel.

Besides, the vast majority of foods and even supplements today actually taste quite good, so having the assumption that they're going to be "bad" doesn't do you any "good" and goes a long way towards preventing you from living a healthier lifestyle. It amazes me how many people will discard the Paleo diet idea because they "don't like any of the food." "There's nothing to eat"! they whine. Give me a break! Anyone who can't find anything they like among meats, vegetables, fruits, good fats and nuts is obviously eating nothing but carbs and junk, and no one should make the assumption that they or their children can live on sodas, potato chips, bread and fast food and achieve or maintain health.

Just open your mind (instead of a bag or box) about food and there are plenty of truly delicious food items to eat. Even snack foods have healthy alternatives available. There is a veritable plethora of cookbooks, websites and even Paleo- compliant-ready-made foods available online. When I first started reducing wheat in 1996, there weren't many alternatives, but there are now. Quit complaining and start looking at the health food store and informational websites for healthier, and might I add, tastier alternatives.

Choosing and Taking the "Right" Supplements

Probably the most obvious difference in the way I work (or so I'm told) is that I don't believe in the necessity or benefit of taking a lot of supplements. Everything that goes into your body, whether it's a fast food burger or CoQ10, must pass through your body's filters. And if your liver gets tired, you're going to get tired. While lecturing in Nashville once, a woman proudly boasted to me that she was taking 52 different supplements. Before I could stop myself, the "Are you *crazy*?" hurled from my mouth. Honestly, how does she think her liver feels about 52 supplements a day? Poor thing; my heart went out to her liver. Just digesting the gel caps alone must be a body burden.

I generally put people on a program of supplements that detoxifies the roadblocks to health (metals, Candida, parasites, etc.), then hope to have them maintain wellness with only four primary things: Immune system support, enzymes (I have my own "house blend" formulated for me), sufficient water, and the Spectrum Balance® or other Paleo/grain-free diet. Generally speaking, if a person still has all his or her organs, then this is usually all they need.

As for vitamins and minerals, here's a thought: *EAT* them, don't take them. If you eat good quality foods that are also the *right* foods, and take enzymes, then generally you won't need to take loads of dietary supplements including vitamins and minerals. But for this to be true, all those steps are required. If you want to eat the wrong foods and skip the enzymes, then you will need to supplement with vitamins. A lot of them. But don't forget to keep detoxing your filters from time to time. All those gel caps you know...

The other danger of taking too many supplements at the same time is what I refer to as "vitamin stacking." Many of these products have been formulated to be "full spectrum" and therefore supposed to be taken alone, so when you start taking too many multi-nutrients together you run the risk of reaching toxicity levels. Granted, not many vitamins, herbals, etc. even *have* a recognized toxicity level, but some fat-soluble ones like Vitamin A and Vitamin E for example, do. The rest, like Vitamins C and B's, will just flush out of your body instead of becoming toxic (ever seen that incredibly neon-yellow urine while taking supplements?), and that still seems like a ridiculous waste of money to me at best.

Often this situation arises when people are taking a particular "line" of products that they may even be representing through a home distribution business or otherwise. They start out using one or two, and pretty soon they're taking a ton of them because they want to try more and more of the product line. If a little is good, then a lot is better, right? Wrong. Do yourself a favor – Go get all your supplements and line them up together. I'll wait here...

OK. Now, add up how many milligrams of any given substance you're taking. Surprise! Also notice that almost all of these products say that they are "full spectrum," "complete," or they are "providing 100%" (or close to it) of the daily requirements (known now as "DV/Daily Value"). This means that if you're taking too many of these, then some substances may likely be accumulating to toxic or near toxic levels. Too much of a good thing, literally! (Note: Add up your "manganese" supplementation before reading Chapter 12). That's why having a supplement program designed for you by your Naturopath or other health care provider who is trained in such things is a great idea. We're here to make sure you're getting enough, but not too much, of nutrients beyond your foods. But even if you don't have an advisor, at least do the math.

Enzymes are mentioned above and I'm going to do it again. And I'll probably do it again and again until you dream about enzymes just from reading this book. I'm a monster on enzymes.

Most people just associate them with digestion actions, but there are actually several different types of enzymes: Digestive, metabolic, antioxidant and systemic, and you need a broad spectrum of them. Enzymes are required for just about every process in your body, but are especially important for digestion, absorption and regulating inflammation. Quite a few people have told me that they don't have much money for supplements, but they do take a multivitamin. If you want my advice; if you can only afford one thing, take a good-quality enzyme instead.

Taking fewer supplements also helps in another way – your budget. A lot of people just don't have enough disposable income to take a fistful of supplements three times a day. True, some would say, "Isn't your health the most important thing? Isn't that where you should spend the most money?" There's a lot of truth to that. It's a bit sanctimonious and annoying perhaps, but true. While I think supplements are usually more important than spending money on jewelry or new aluminum rims for your truck, for a lot of folks it isn't so much a choice between a trip to Cancun or supplements, it's more like a choice between paying the rent, or putting gas in the car, or supplements. And let's get real; the best supplement in the world isn't going to do much for you if you don't have a roof over your head!

And last, taking fewer supplements is vital in the most important part of my protocols – compliance. If you ask most people to carry around a bag of supplements with them at all times, and take a whole bunch of stuff three or even more times a day, it just isn't going to happen! Maybe some practitioners can get people to do that, but it hasn't been my experience. I don't personally like taking a bunch of pills, so it's easy for me to understand why others would feel the same way.

Time Frame

Also helpful budget-wise is that as a general rule, I don't tend to see people on a long-term basis, unless of course their specific conditions warrant it. Most commonly I see someone once a month for only three to six months (travel permitting), then ask him or her to check in once a year after that. I don't see the point in having an appointment once a month just for me to say, "Okay, keep doing what you're doing." So, if it's just a matter of taking maintenance supplements, sticking to their diet, drinking plenty of water and exercising, I cut them loose on their own recognizance pretty quickly. Natural medicine after all, is *lifestyle medicine*, and is best maintained with one's lifestyle, not endless office visits.

This also means that I usually have room to take on new clients. Note: If you call a Naturopath's office and they say they aren't taking new clients? Well... you probably don't want to go there anyway. If a Naturopath is efficient and routinely releasing clients, then they should have openings. That's all I'm saying.

Many other Naturopaths have asked me how I get my clients to be so compliant, and this is the bottom line. I ask my clients to take a few very important things, and/or have them add things in stages so there's not so much to do at once. I would rather recommend fewer supplements and have people take them, than recommend everything they could possibly need and they don't take any. As I tell clients all the time, the supplements work better on the *inside*. They need to make their way out of the bottles and into your body in order to do their work.

Education

As important as detoxification and supplements are, the most important element of my program is education. I spend a lot of time educating people about food additives and where they lurk. I don't tell them to exercise, I tell them *why* to exercise and how modest exercise works with their bodily systems for their health. Instead of lecturing them on drinking water, I explain the extremely detrimental effects of dehydration on every aspect of their bodies and give them easy-to-do tips on getting into the habit of drinking more water and getting it to absorb better in their bodies.

Most important, I work with each person individually to adopt healthy eating, exercising and other practices *within his or her unique lifestyle*. No two people have the same schedule, so sometimes you have to figure a way around it. For example, one of my clients is a missionary who travels so much that she doesn't even have her own apartment. We figured out what she could eat in airports, and how to gently get the people she stayed with to understand that there is more to life than meatloaf and mashed potatoes. Because we worked *with* her lifestyle instead of trying to change it, she has managed to regain her health and vitality and lose more than sixty pounds in the process.

One of the hardest things I do, and I do try hard, is to get people to have realistic expectations about their health goals. As this varies greatly from person to person it is a bit tough to explain, but I'll try. If people with all their organs are willing to take the small, reasonable amount of supplements they really need, eat what they should eat, drink enough water and get some exercise than they can expect an optimum result from their bodies.

Then the subtractions begin, or as I think of it, you start trying to walk *up* the down escalator. If you are unwilling to do one or more of the things listed above, start subtracting. If you are missing organs, subtract again. If you are taking prescription drugs, especially those with substantial side effects, subtract some more. For example, I had a woman who, after we got her blood sugar and blood pressure sorted out and she felt significantly better, wanted to know why she still (there's that "still" again) didn't have more energy. I told her to ask her doctor about the *five* anti-depressants she was taking as all five carried the PDR-listed side effect of "fatigue." If you and your doctor make the decision that you need to be on five tranquilizers, *and who knows, maybe you do*, then you need to realistically expect some fatigue. That's what I mean by being realistic. I'm a Naturopath, not a magician.

As tolerant as I try to be, I do have my "bottom lines", although not always the ones people expect. Several people have flinched back for cover when telling me that they smoke, expecting I think, for me to throw some sort of fit and hit them over the head with a pig bladder or something. Instead I usually start by telling them to first switch to an all-natural tobacco cigarette. The reasons for this are twofold; for one thing, natural tobacco is substantially less detrimental to your health than the chemicals added to most cigarettes, and also because natural tobacco is much easier to quit using. That's why cigarette companies put the additives in there in the first place; to keep cigarettes from going out if you stop puffing on it (can't have you lighting up the same butt twice – less profit), and to keep you addicted.

People used to quit too often and too easily before some geniuses poured in the additives – seems quitting is really bad for business. *Note to the gentlemen: Do you know what is commonly used to keep the cigarette burning when you lay it down? Salt peter. Maybe that will shed some new light on some of your issues right there.* So if you start people off by switching brands, they get to keep the habit, but lose their addiction to the chemicals. *Then* they can quit much easier when they only have the habit to break and not the combo with the chemical addiction. We've created a lot of non-smokers using this system. Again, working *with* their lifestyles is the right way to go.

However, there are areas where I pull no punches. I'm usually okay with people cutting down by increments on soda and coffee consumption (although I am more adamant about sodas), but I reach a full stop when it comes to diet sodas. None. Zero. Zip. Not even one. I would rather watch people drink insecticide...oh, wait! That's what they're already doing! Some artificial sweeteners, lest it slip your mind, are neurotoxins originally created to be ant poison. Look it up for yourself.

My other blind spot is water. Most people are chronically dehydrated, and there is a laundry list of symptoms that will not go away if you remain dehydrated. I will be talking more about these issues later in the book, so I will leave them here for now.

So, to recap the basics of your program:
1. Organ/ filter detoxification <u>first</u>
2. Identifying and detoxing your "roadblocks" to health
3. Immune system boosters/modulators and enzymes

4. Good *quality* food that are also the *right* foods
5. Drinking sufficient pure water

This is the foundation that everything else I do is built upon. Every one of the thousands we've worked with started with those same five simple practices. It's amazing what can be accomplished when you start in this very simple and straightforward way.

Getting My Points Across

As you've probably already noticed, I use a lot of metaphors and analogies in my work. I think that often a simple comparison is the fastest and most easily understandable way to make your point with people. Unless I'm lecturing, I usually only have an hour or less to convey a tremendous amount of information. So if I sound like a TV sports announcer from time to time please forgive me. I used to sometimes worry about this lack of syllables on my part, until a while back when three different people said essentially the same thing on the same day.

I like the first one of the day the best, so I'll quote her. She said, "Shauna, you have never said a medical sounding word to me, and I love it. If I can get it, I can do it. And I'm getting well because of it, against what all the Latin-spewers said." This works for me. I've heard many names used to describe allopaths, but "Latin-spewers" was a new one on me. For the record; I know very little Latin, but I'm working on my Italian.

CHAPTER 3

Allopath vs. Naturopath

"Our figures show approximately four and one half million hospital admissions annually due to the adverse reactions to drugs. Further the average hospital patient has as much as a thirty percent chance, depending on how long he is in, of doubling his stay due to adverse drug reactions."

— Milton Silverman, M.D. Prof.
of Pharmacology, University of California

Let me be extremely and unquestionably clear on this: We greatly need MD's and I am definitely *not* anti-MD. For instance, don't come to me with your broken bones – I'd have no clue, and I have no desire to have a clue on those kinds of problems. In fact, let me state for the record here that I have the utmost respect for many doctors, especially ER docs. There is a whole wealth of procedures that an MD can perform that I cannot. I'm truly very happy where I am, thank you very much. However, having said this let me also say that I think that there is not only room, but a *need* for both kinds of doctors – Allopathic and Naturopathic.

I feel for MD's, I really do. For one thing, most of them are probably not practicing the way they really want, but are instead practicing based on rigidly applied standards of patient care and the demands and expectations of their patients for instant gratification! They have to wade around in blood and guts (and worse), they have to take mountains of crap from insurance companies and HMOs (I've seen a few good doctors quit because of the HMO demands), they pay horrendous malpractice insurance costs, and they have to wear white coats. I personally don't look good in white, and opt to wear much nicer clothes to work – a definite perk. And the worst part: Medical doctors almost always see you when you're already sick. Not that I don't see my share of sick people, but my primary job is to try to keep my clients from getting that way in the first place.

Before we get too far into this, let me clarify the terms. Some of these are broad generalizations and certainly aren't representative of all Allopaths or all Naturopaths, but it will give you a place to start.

An Allopath is a medical doctor, an "M.D." An Allopath's extensive training is in cataloging symptoms of illness in order to diagnose diseases, then treating those diseases primarily through surgery, drugs or radiation, ergo the "cut, poison and burn" mentality. MD's receive very little training about diet and nutrition, as most medical schools do not consider them to be important factors. They often do painful, humiliating and invasive testing procedures like x-rays, MRI's, biopsies and the like in order to make a diagnosis. Generally speaking (apart from regular physical exams), they wait for you to get sick and then attempt to treat or mitigate the symptoms; in other words *reactive* medicine. Allopaths generally consider that as long as you're doing okay in keeping your symptoms in check using medications, that you're "healthy." They are addressed as "Dr. (Whomever)" (it amazes me how many people do not even know their doctors' first names), and the people they treat are referred to as their "patients."

A Naturopath is a natural medicine doctor, an "N.D." which stands for "Naturopathic Doctor," or this week for me, a "C.T.N." which is a "Certified Traditional Naturopath." Next week I suppose I might have to be referred to as a "P.W.H.S.F.D.I.A.H.", or "Person Who Has Some Fairly Decent Ideas About Health", for all I know. Honestly, this havoc over titles is exhausting! Our training, which is rather extensive, is in general wellness, boosting the immune system to prevent dis-ease, and in finding natural ways without harmful side effects to work with symptoms that have already developed. We use no invasive testing procedures.

We try to restore people to a state of glowing, radiant health, and do not consider doing "okay" or being maintained on perpetual drugs as "health." In contrast to the primarily reactive nature of allopathic medicine, we would define naturopathic medicine as predominantly *proactive*.

Although a few of the more adventurous have called me things like "Doc Sky" (my initials and email address), or "Dr. Shauna" and one lovely lady from Kansas calls me "Sis" (which is my personal favorite), I am generally referred to as "Shauna" and the people I see are "clients", a term I have no problem with since very few of those I would be calling "patients" have much *patience* anyway. Of course some of the doctors in the area have come up with a few more names for me, but I don't want to offend anyone so I won't include them here.

Sick Care vs. Health Care

A huge difference between Allopaths and Naturopaths is that Allopaths are trained to fix what's already broken, while Naturopaths are trained to help prevent it from being broken in the first place: Fixing versus preventing, and treating symptoms versus identifying and addressing the root causes.

Allopaths and Naturopaths have virtually nothing in common. To paraphrase an architect of the 1994 Dietary Supplement Health and Education Act (DSHEA), we have both a "sick care system" and a "health care system." Can you guess who does what?

However, Allopaths and Naturopaths both have a desire to see people get well, and we both use our training to the best of our abilities to make that happen. We just have very little common ground in doing it. That's why this recent trend in so-called "Integrated Medicine" is so jumbled to me. It's like thinking that you can continue to be on the fast-food/nicotine/aspartame diet and somehow still be healthy. It's a convenient theory, but I wouldn't give you a snowball's chance of it working! There needs to be some actual Naturopaths in on this process to really "integrate" it, and that is exceedingly rare.

From what I can tell, this trend in *integrating* is mostly coming because the public is far more interested than ever in using natural supplements, the trend continues to grow, and their doctors don't want to lose patients to Naturopaths who actually specialize in the proper use of dietary supplements. While coming back from a training session in Cancun, I read in the airline magazine that a "major medical study" had just concluded that "vitamins were good for you." Gee, no kidding. They call this *integration*? All I know is that in school, if you copied off someone else's paper, they didn't call it "integration"!

Frankly, most of what I've seen of integration is doctors who still want to do surgery, radiation and drugs, but they also suggest use of some Vitamin C as well. Some integration. It doesn't give me a lot of faith in their desire and belief in "integrating". And quite honestly, I just don't see much positive result in my people who have tried to integrate to that extent. So basically, Integrated Medicine is no more than a *marketing* term to try to convince people that all options will be on the table and available to them.

I encourage people to do careful and extensive research, get opinions from people they trust, give it mindful consideration, then pick the side they are comfortable with and stick to it one hundred percent. If you feel most comfortable with surgery or chemo, then do exactly as your doctor says with no deviations. If you want to go with the natural approach, then jump in with both feet while holding your water bottle. But you've got to do it *all* the way, and most important, **you need to believe in it totally.** It's tough to get well any other way.

Vital information to understand: With most illnesses but particularly with cancer, which is the one that gets "integrated" the most, any truly *aggressive* Allopathic or Naturopathic protocols not only may not work *with* one another, but may likely work *against* one another. Case in point: Chemo is intended to *defeat* your immune system, while supplement regimes will be intended to *maximize* your immune system. As I've said before, it's like walking up a descending escalator – you don't get anywhere! Please note that I said "truly aggressive" on this. There are many, many supplements that can help curb the damage caused by treatments such as radiation or chemo, for example taking a therapeutic dose of CoQ10 can help keep your heart healthy while undergoing radiation treatments, but those are *complementary* – not aggressive.

There is a vast difference between supplements designed to help prevent damage, and ones that are aggressively targeting a dis-ease. The aggressive ones *do not complement* one another. And you would be hard pressed to find a Naturopath who would find *any* good coming from weakening your immune system, which is the basis of chemo.

Finally, the biggest stumbling block to "integration" in my opinion is that any available "middle ground" is really getting trampled. Why? Because the practitioners *on both sides of the issue* are not truly open to working together because the schools of thought are so far apart. Why do we need to separate into these camps of such extremes with the camps getting farther and farther apart by the day? The Allopathic group is now often perceived as a knife-wielding, drug riddled, hardcore group of robots, which is preposterous, while the Naturopathic group is thought of as a bunch of crystal waving, incense burning, leaf eaters, which is just as crazy! It is this extremity of opinion that is truly dangerous and singularly prevents the use of the best from both worlds for the good of the client/patient in question.

Naturopaths are huge targets for oversight and regulation, which is quite strange since according to JAMA (*Journal of the American Medical Association*), medical doctors (MD's) are the number-one cause of death in the U.S.! Yep, it's called "Iatrogenic deaths," which translates to "physician caused." Heart disease and cancer have taken the number two and three slots respectively. One recent JAMA study attributed 2,036,884 unnecessary deaths *per year* directly to the American medical system, and shows a whopping $122 billion yearly in "unnecessary procedures".

Although I couldn't find a specific statistic for this, I would be willing to bet that more people are killed annually by things like lightning or goat stampedes than any deaths attributed to seeing

Traditional Naturopaths. So why are <u>we</u> under the microscope? Certainly one reason is because Naturopaths do not fit anywhere in the AMA's "Usual and Customary Standards of Practice", and the AMA has a long history of shutting down anyone who can't be pigeon-holed into its standards. In other words, anyone who is not an MD.

Just to enable me to practice, I am compelled by law to put this statement into all my client intake paperwork:

"This practitioner does not practice the application of scientific principles to prevent, diagnose, and treat physical and mental diseases, disorders and conditions or to safeguard the health of any woman and infant through pregnancy and parturition."

Why anyone would even care what I thought after signing such a document is a testimony to the strength of the referral he or she got to come to me in the first place! "Not practicing the application of scientific principles"? Do they want people to think I'm just pulling all this stuff out of my... hat? In there with the monkeys I suppose.

In China, they have what they call "Barefoot Doctors". These people have herbal as opposed to standard medical training, so they are more like ND's than MD's. They are assigned to villages, not to treat people if they get sick, but rather to keep everyone healthy and therefore working and productive. A Medical Doctor goes out of business if no one gets sick, while a Barefoot Doctor gets fired if *too many* people get sick. Two different purposes, and yet they work very well together in China, and both are respected. How come we can't do that?

As I've told many of my clients, I am much more related to these "Barefoot Doctors" or to one of those Appalachian old ladies who live at the edge of the holler' who can "make a tea" for whatever ails you, than to *anyone* in a white coat. This is one reason that the notion of not always being addressed as "Doctor Young" (despite my PhD) doesn't particularly bug me. The difference is I'm not interested in putting *them* out of business! I also don't call them "quacks" or other intentionally unfavorable appellations. And it's a good thing I don't have that particular inclination, since I could get arrested if I do!

Which brings us to another charming law. Doctors can say anything they want about a natural practitioner, and it is considered to be their "medical opinion". There is a doctor here in my town that has actually (according to these people) told clients of mine that "they're lucky I haven't killed them"! The fact that he has zero basis for this statement, and only mutters darkly when asked to elaborate on it, means nothing. And although several of my irritated clients have offered to testify in court that he states these and other atrocities against me with regularity, my lawyer informs me that there is nothing to be done about it. This doctor even put forth some of this same nonsense (accidentally) to a friend of mine *at a medical convention*, and there is still no recourse for me to stop him. The only way I could go after him at all is if I could prove he hurts my business, and since all these people still see me, there is no provable basis for that. He hasn't hurt me, he just ticks me off. And there is no legal "cease and desist" for being ticked off.

Naturopaths on the other hand, are prevented by law from criticizing or challenging anything an Allopath says or does so that the authority of the medical doctor is not undermined; undermined authority being a very big deal to these folks. As one of my clients asked of her MD when he expressed that she was unnecessarily questioning his opinion/authority, "When did you being right become more important than my health?" Good point. Someone could walk into my office with a scalpel actually protruding from his forehead, and if I said that I didn't think it was a good idea for his surgeon to have left it there, I could be in real trouble. I think this is one reason that I'm always teetering on the edge of TMJ. Sometimes it's hard to keep your mouth shut, so you clamp it shut.

Philosophies Apart

Your classic conventional doctor tends to focus largely on addressing symptoms; generally with the use of drugs and/or surgery.

Common medical procedure is less about investigating or identifying the underlying causes of symptoms, but instead may be content with maintaining control over symptoms using artificial drugs that most patients have to stay on for long periods of time or even for a lifetime. As Naturopaths, we try to find reasons and causes behind the symptoms and then remove the *causes* for the condition by natural means, including detoxification or supplementation. That's a big difference right there. As an example, most Allopaths do not consider environmental causes behind illness like artificial food additives, hazardous workplaces and radiation. Naturopaths specialize in them.

Further, Allopaths do not generally recognize the concept of ever being "healed". For example, once your doctor puts you on thyroid, blood pressure or cholesterol medication, he or she usually expects you to be on it for life, even if the symptoms go away. As more people adopt healthier lifestyle habits, this can be very problematic health wise.

For example, I worked with a woman taking blood pressure medication who with our help completely changed her diet and lifestyle. Since she was still taking a beta-blocker, her blood pressure had dropped to a dangerously low level where she was cold, tired and dizzy all the time, and her doctor *still* didn't want her off that medication! He was concerned that her hypertension might return. Since, as a Naturopath, I can't suggest she stop taking any medication, I was instead trying to give her some advice on how to raise her blood pressure until she could get in to see a new doctor. She showed her sense of humor by saying, "I know what to do. All the stuff I've been told *not* to do for the last 15 years!"

More than ever, Allopaths believe in "pre" conditions and, of course, in medicating them; "pre-diabetic", "pre-hypertensive", "pre-cancerous", etc. If it's "pre", then doesn't that mean that the condition doesn't exist yet? I ski, so does that mean I'm "pre-broken leg" and should start wearing a cast and take Percoset for the pain that will surely come? In my mind this "pre" thing and the idea of leaping to medicating *numbers* as opposed to actual *symptoms* is really getting misunderstood and out of hand.

And how do physicians even keep up? Take the *Merck Manual* for example. My first *Merck Manual* is only a few years old and yet tons of the guidelines are already outdated. As one example, the "acceptable" numbers for blood sugar, TSH, blood pressure, cholesterol and multiple others continue to be skewed lower and lower, which then includes an ever-widening section of the public. A cynical person would say that this is one reason why there are so many more prescriptions being written for these conditions, but after all, we hear that it's all done in the name of being "safer". A vast majority of people are now having these "elevated" (read *"lowered"*) numbers "discovered" during routine physicals, and although they have no adverse symptoms from this "problem" they are put immediately on medication to keep one from occurring.

Interesting. Because more and more of these people are winding up in offices like mine wondering why they feel worse than they did before their doctors had a numeric "discovery"! Side effects my friends, side effects. Despite the fact that my blood pressure has been essentially the same since I was thirteen years old (in fact it's slightly lower now), it is now considered by the new standards to be in the "borderline high" or "pre-hypertension" area and therefore I guess I'm ripe to be medicated. Being that I've had it for almost 40 years with no problems doesn't seem to count for much! After that length of time, it seems more "post" than "pre" to me, don't you think?

Allopaths are also okay with using drugs for maintenance. Naturopaths, however, stress *change* – the right foods, enough water and exercise, and getting rid of the patterns and habits that caused the symptoms in the first place. Doesn't taking a pill to relieve a symptom only reinforce the bad habit that caused the problem in the first place? Yes!

Admittedly, taking the pills is a lot easier than changing your diet or getting yourself off the couch, but the side effects can be as bad as what you're taking them for in the first place. Look in the trusty, aforementioned PDR or listen more closely to the rapid-fire disclosures at the end of drug ads on TV if you don't believe me. And I can tell you from experience that the side effects of good diet and exercise are very pleasant.

Another typical problem working with Allopaths can be one of communication. Most doctors do not like being questioned. A bewildering amount of my clients have been discharged by their doctors for asking too many questions like, "Why do you want me to take this?" or, "What are the side effects of this?" Most Naturopaths are very open to such questions, and I personally encourage my clients to investigate my theories on their own and to do *independent* research.

This brings up another important point: I find it interesting that a vast predominance of the "informational" websites doctors refer to are sponsored and/or provided by drug companies! I recently performed my own investigation out of curiosity. I logged onto a depression support website and although I filled out the online questionnaire about six different ways (with symptoms of six different conditions) it always came to the conclusion that I was severely depressed and recommended that I immediately start taking the company's pill. Big shocker.

Doctors "diagnose" diseases, and come up with names for them. Naturopaths, however, see diseases as "dis-*ease*" and view them just as groups of symptoms that have causes. We don't need to name them, we just need to figure out the cause (or causes) and get rid of them. Why would anyone want a disease named after him or her anyway? Personally, I would hate to have someone suffering from some hideous condition and use my name to describe it! Baseball legend Lou Gehrig was a very talented athlete and from all accounts, a helluva guy, but his athletic prowess is somewhat overshadowed by the disease named after him. I mean, is that really any way to celebrate a legend?

Blinded by Studies

Now the main reason why I would *never* want to be an MD is that they perform and/or take part in double-blind testing. The vast majority of Naturopaths could not live with ourselves if we did, which is why we don't.

Since we don't, all of our evidence and data is considered "anecdotal", while the Allopathic results are "empirical." No problem, I'll take it. No one has to die to get anecdotal evidence. Medicine is supposed to be an art and a science, each balancing the other. In my mind this obsessive need for empirical evidence using double-blind testing removes any "art" involved and just leaves cold-blooded science. The idea of knowingly giving a placebo to a sick and dying person when you think the drug could save them is the stuff of nightmares for me.

A few years ago a woman with a severe liver disease came into my office. The minute she confessed that she was in a clinical trial I immediately stopped the consultation, because legally I had to. I told her that I could not work with her at all, that she did not have to pay for the part of the consultation we had already started, and most of all, I wished her luck. Sadly, she knew that she was receiving the placebo and was in great pain and afraid to die. She begged her doctor in the trial to let her out; he wouldn't. They needed the empirical evidence her death would create. She called and begged me to help her. I couldn't because this is the kind of thing that sends Naturopaths to jail. It broke my heart to not help her, but my hands were tied.

Her husband called soon after that to tell me that she had died. He wanted me to know that they didn't blame me for my decision and inability to offer help. Unfortunately it still took me a long time to feel the same way. So, here's the question I would ask Big Pharma and doctors: How would you feel if it was your child, your wife or husband, your Mom or Dad who was getting the placebo? No Naturopath has had to ask themselves that question. Thank goodness.

True Allopathic Colors: Three Case Studies

Admittedly, my own personal experiences with most MD's have not been good. There have been a few cases where they were helpful, even kind, but overwhelmingly in my life the awful has far outweighed the good. A book chronicling even half of the horror stories I've heard from clients over the years would be thousands of pages long, so instead I will include just three examples from my personal collection:

#1: This one has occurred many times, but this particular instance was maybe the most extreme.

While having dinner with some friends one evening and waiting for our table in the bar (yes, I do drink on occasion), a woman I didn't know asked me the inevitable question, "So what do you do for a living?"

My friends rolled their eyes at this, since this question often launches an inquisition. After I told her, she (as usual) asked if she could ask me "one quick question," in this case about anti-depressants. This "one quick question" thing feels at times, like the bane of my existence, as it is never one, and rarely quick. This evening, every time I answered one of her questions, a man a few seats down the bar would snort loudly and derisively. I ignored him, but my inquisitive cocktail companion did not, and finally asked him what he was "snorting about". With a very patronizing look and tone, he informed her that he was "a real doctor", that everything I had told her was complete nonsense, and that people like me "should all be put away".

Being used to this kind of goofy and ignorant abuse, I ignored him, but she didn't. She asked him to tell her specifically what part of what I'd said was untrue. He tried to drown her in generalizations, that "all of it" was ridiculous, that "she wouldn't understand it anyway", etc., but she wasn't buying. She wanted specifics. At this point, I finally joined in. I started with basics: Why do MAOI's (mono amine oxidase inhibitors) contraindicate with so many other drugs and even food? After much hemming and hawing, it turned out that not only did he not know the reasons for the contraindications, he didn't even know what MAOI stands for. I felt a wave of pity for this real doctor's patients. She then asked me for explanations, which I gave her.

Fortunately, the hostess picked this moment to tell us our table was ready, and we left the good doctor to snort in peace with his rum and Diet Coke®. His inquisitor told him she hoped that he'd learn to mind his own business (and his snorts).

#2: I know this one sounds like some kind of a horrible exaggeration, but I swear to you that it's true. This was the day now known forever in my mind with capital letters: The Day I was Dispossessed of My Cheery Notion of All of Us Holding Hands and Working Together.

A few years into practice, I received an invitation from the local hospital to attend a seminar on "Contraindications Between Herbal Remedies and Chemotherapy Drugs". That sounded interesting so I RSVP'd, ASAP.

When I arrived at the lecture, I was surrounded by a sea of white coats and scrubs, not another natural practitioner in sight. No problem. Just some information being given to health practitioners, right? There were no torches or pitchforks in sight, and I had been personally invited. Unfortunately, my cool (and my TMJ) were about to be immediately and forcefully tested.

At first there was a little information I already knew about regarding herbals like St. John's Wort that contraindicate with chemotherapy estrogen site blockers (as they compete for the same sites), but all in all I felt they had left out a lot of others. Just to show you how naive I was I actually had thoughts of approaching the lecturer (an MD) afterward and giving him some info and websites regarding some others! These happy thoughts of mutual professional enlightenment were banished quickly as minutes later it became clear what this lecture was *really* about. The real title should have been, "How Not to Lose Business to Natural Practitioners".

He explained that Naturopaths were a danger since "natural types" are very "touchy-feely" with people, sometimes going so far as to hug them, which people like, and giving them "a feeling of being cared about". He further suggested to the note-taking crowd that they do things like "be sure to look at the chart before going in to make sure you know the patient's name" like natural practitioners do, that they stand in front of the mirror to "practice looking compassionate", to learn "how to compose their faces and not look judgmental when people want to talk about their vitamins" and that it was "better to talk them out of their supplements while seeming to care about them". And every time he mentioned a natural practitioner, he would put up a specific picture on his overhead projector that drew derisive and indulgent chuckles from the crowd; a duck with a stethoscope around its neck. Talk about a "spin" doctor!

Anyway, by now I was grinding my teeth so hard that my head was pounding! "*Pretend* to care about your patients?" "*Practice* looking compassionate"? Who *is* this guy and what planet did he come from? And the truly alarming thing was that no one seemed unduly upset except me. All these doctors sitting around me were just nodding and taking notes. Where *was* I, in the freaking Twilight Zone? Part of me wanted to jump up and run, but I was frozen to my chair like someone looking at an auto accident or something. It was grisly, but I couldn't look away.

The lecture ended and I thought I'd be released from my prison, but no. A question-and-answer period was next. Based on the questions they were asking, I couldn't believe these people were actually in the health care industry! All I could think of at this point was "Shauna, escape!" when suddenly I realized that the "quack of some sort" who was being derided by an oncologist behind me, was actually me! She was warning everyone about losing patients to these quacks, because she had lost several to me, mostly because "They seem to think she cares about them or is invested in their health or something." The lecturer asked if the particular patient she had discussed had gotten any good out of my treatments, and she said she "didn't know". Okay, that's it. No more.

Rising (I hope) with grace, I informed the white-coated and scrub-bedecked audience that first of all I had been invited to this fiasco and therefore wasn't gate-crashing, then I introduced myself to the crowd, gesturing at his oh-so-funny picture on the overhead and identifying myself as the "quack" in question.

Next I confronted the oncologist, who was currently trying to slide under the table. I asserted that she knew exactly what happened to the patient under discussion, and why didn't she tell everyone else? The lecturer asked her what she knew, and she sat there mute. So he asked me.

The reason the woman had came to me in the first place was because this doctor had given up on her, told her to "Go home and get her affairs in order." In other words, die. She didn't care much for that option and came to me hoping for another. Six months had passed since then, and she was still hanging in there. The complete lack of response from the doctor confirmed to them all that what I'd just said was true. That shut the room up. I picked up my things to leave, but couldn't resist two parting shots: I told the room at large that the day I had to fake compassion would be my last as a health practitioner, and I told the oncologist to be more careful about bad-mouthing people, especially someone who might be in the room.

It took me a long time to get over this debacle; it just seemed too unreal. I did however get one gift from this lecture. The picture the lecturer put up every time he mentioned a natural practitioner was certainly meant to be an insult, but I didn't take it that way. Instead, I embraced it. His insult has become my symbol.

#3: This is a personal one, but from listening to client accounts, I'm far from the only person who has had similar experiences.

Because of a free HMO policy I had through a place I previously worked, I had to get "routine" tests from time to time. This time it was a PAP test. I came home on a Friday night and got a message on my answering machine from the doctor's office. Apparently there was "something wrong" with my PAP test, and I needed to call the doctor "ASAP on Monday". She then wished me a "good weekend". Fat chance. I think I manifested about 150 symptoms that weekend just from thinking about it!

First thing on Monday I called. The office administrator told me the doctor wanted to speak with me in person and made an appointment for me – ten days away. Ten days? Couldn't I just talk to him on the phone? Get a hint of some kind? No deal.

Ten hideous days later, I went in for my appointment. The doctor came in, opened my chart, and without ever once looking at me he started in. As I sat there frozen with shock he explained in a completely unemotional voice that according to my test, I was in Stage 4 cervical and ovarian cancer. I would need an immediate hysterectomy, followed by chemo and radiation treatments, but he still didn't want me to "hold out too much hope" that I would live despite the treatments. He closed the chart, and looked at me for the first time. "I'm sorry *Amanda*", he said.

It took me a minute to realize what he'd said, but when I found my voice, I croaked, "Who is Amanda?" He looked at me in surprise. "*You* are. Amanda Young." When I told him that no, I was *Shauna* Young, he thought I was "in denial". I had to show the idiot my driver's license! His response? "Oh. Well never mind", and he got up and left. *Never mind*? After I'd been through nearly two weeks (and the last 15 minutes) of hell? I staggered out of his office and laid down on the grass in the parking lot, trying not to throw up.

Right then and there I swore that was *never* going to happen to me again, and I'd do my best to ensure that it didn't happen to others either. The vague ideas of Naturopathic school that had been flitting around in my brain were now getting clearer. Not only had I been put through the ringer, but what about poor Amanda? Two weeks had passed in her dire situation while they messed around with the wrong person!

A week later the doctor's office called. They couldn't find my PAP test and wanted me to come in for another. No thanks. I have to give them credit for nerve, though.

As I stated before, there are more differences than common ground between Allopaths and Naturopaths, but we do have one thing in common. You. We both want you to get well. It is up to you to decide what kind of care you are most comfortable with and then get completely behind it.

Before we move along to the next chapter, there's one last question in this whole Allopath/Naturopath realm that bugs me: Why are *we* considered "alternative"? While modern "western medicine" is relatively new, the form of medicine I practice is as old as mankind itself. There is evidence of herbs being used medicinally all the way back to Neanderthals, and the extremely well preserved "Ice Man" they found in Switzerland (a Cro-Magnon) had some of the very same mushrooms in his possession that I use for health purposes today. If we need all these modern drugs to survive, then how did mankind make it all these years without them?

Alternative? I don't think so.

CHAPTER 4

Naturopath vs. Naturopath

"Can't we all just get along?"
— RODNEY KING

Please don't skip this little chapter. You may not feel that this subject applies to you, but it does. It has to do with your rights and freedom of choice regarding health care. It's short, but it's vitally important. While an entire book could be written on this particular issue, I don't want to spend that much time with it, and in fact I'm going to be very brief. However there is a little known battle taking place; one that represents a tremendous threat to your health choices and freedoms and definitely warrants some attention and concern.

Although not widely known, it is often not medical doctors giving Traditional Naturopaths the most problems, but rather other Naturopathic organizations, primarily the AANP (American Association of Naturopathic Physicians). A different version of Naturopaths who believe that they are "more qualified" due to their particular educational profile and should therefore be the only ones allowed to be *licensed* to practice, or at least that's the official party line. I think it has a lot more to do with money than concerns for public safety. What do Traditional Naturopaths do at any rate that could cause someone *harm*? As I once jokingly told a client that since all the supplements and everything else I work with are natural, "If I really didn't like you I guess I could give you a case of diarrhea." It's an oversimplification, but very close to the reality.

When a State considers "licensing" natural medicine, it may seem to many like it would be a positive thing if one is under the assumption that the regulatory process will somehow "allow" or better "legitimize" natural practitioners. But the reality is that it is simply an opportunity to create a professional and financial monopoly for only a select group of Naturopaths – a type of doctor incidentally that is vastly outnumbered by the practitioners they are attempting to disallow, which are primarily under the ANMA, ANCB and NTCB associations that have certified Traditional Naturopaths. The AANP is making legislative successes State by State that mandate that unless you attend/attended one of a mere handful of schools (there are only five such schools in the U.S. and two in Canada), you can't practice or even continue to practice as a Naturopath.

Such exclusionary licensing has resulted in making both traditional naturopathy and holistic nutritional counseling *felony* violations of law. And what in reality these lovely sounding laws have resulted in, is in throwing competent, conscientious and caring doctors virtually instantly out of practice with absolutely no "grandfather" rights or even proficiency provisions, leaving the clients they may have been assisting for years or even decades without their trusted advisors.

A dramatic example of this happened to a Naturopath I met from Florida who told me his story of living in a newly licensed State. He was not even aware that Florida had passed a license law. One day he recalled, law enforcement came busting into his office and just shut it down. He was taken to jail and put in a holding cell while his client files were ransacked and confiscated as if he were a common criminal. Far from being grandfathered as should rightly be afforded to honest citizens and legitimate business owners, he was prevented from even one more day of practice. He and his family had to move to another State where he was able to set up shop once again. Fortunately for them, many of his more than 1,000 clients were able to travel to see him at his new location. To know the status of your own State, you can log onto the American Naturopathic Medical Association website at www.anma.org and refer to the national map found there.

So why is this happening? Well, the "Naturopathic Physician" or "N.P." group is looking for a lot of things that Traditional Naturopaths simply do not seek. However, as long as there is a *choice* for the public between more than one type of natural medicine, the NP's see it as a threat to their well-being and authority, not to mention their finances (sounds kind of familiar, doesn't it? Didn't George Orwell capture this tendency in "Animal Farm"?). For one thing, NP's desire to become primary care physicians who are able to collect medical insurance and this is something that most Traditional Naturopaths (including myself) have absolutely no interest in. NP's also want to prescribe drugs and even do minor surgical procedures; something Traditional Naturopaths would avoid like…, well…, drugs and surgery! (You might re-read the definition of "Naturopathy" in the beginning of this book)

It seems to me that if you want to practice with drugs and surgery then you should go to medical school and become an Allopathic Doctor. It seems very strange to me that the same practices that this group embraces, which make them consider themselves *superior* to Traditional Naturopaths, are the very things that make traditionalists consider them *not* to be Naturopaths! They seem more like "wanna-be MD's" stuck somewhere in the middle. Not "integrating" exactly, but rather just not fully qualified on either side of the Allopathic/Naturopathic divide.

Having said that; *please be clear that our traditional side is making no such attempts to see the AANP doctors outlawed from practicing.* Unlike them, we're just fine with people being offered more choices. It is only them trying to stop us as we provide what they perceive as *too much* choice, because it presents challenges to their monopolistic goals. I fully believe that people are fully capable of making their own choices as to what type of practitioner they want to see, consistent with their fundamental and constitutional rights.

The bottom line is: Find a practitioner who gives you what *you* want. If you want some nutritional advice and supplements mixed together with the option of drugs and surgery, then choose a Naturopathic Physician. If you *only* want the advice about *only* natural therapies like food, lifestyle, nutraceuticals and herbals then seek out a Traditional Naturopath. *Just don't try doing this if you live in a licensed State since your "choice" has already been made for you!*

Speaking for myself, I know that many of my clients are very happy seeing a traditionalist that lacks both the desire or capability of ordering tons of blood work, diagnostic testing, x-rays or cutting off little pieces, because they are fully and completely sick of all that. For people who feel they been scammed, abused or harmed by conventional western medicine, the last thing they want to hear is that I think they need to have more tests, surgery or drugs. Thanks, but no thanks. I say leave the drugs and surgery to the MD's.

How Naturopathic Physicians have been able to get a growing number of States to succumb to the license laws is a lot easier to explain. Collectively, they have a lot more money than does our side. I don't know where my dues money to the American Naturopathic Medical Association (ANMA) has gone, but it certainly didn't seem to result in protection of practitioners' rights. While I was a member, I saw the ANMA consistently prove themselves to be a bunch of paper tigers that didn't actually do anything that I can put my finger on, and instead have "compromised" us almost out of existence. The national and State chapters of the Coalition for Natural Health make solid attempts, but they just don't have the big bucks backing them that the AANP and its schools have.

Just as laws and regulations don't enable monopolies for cable television providers or phone companies, they shouldn't be allowed to restrict public access to valuable health care options like Naturopathy. Don't allow important rights and freedom of choice for your health to be taken from you without a vote or a fight.

CHAPTER 5

The Making of a Naturopath

"The doctor of the future will give no medication, but will interest his patients in the care of the human frame, diet, and in the cause and prevention of disease."

— THOMAS A. EDISON

The portion of this chapter that is about the actual required schooling and technical aspects of my chosen profession will be fairly brief. After all, you can find all that on the Internet if you so desire. What I'm going to mostly address here is what it takes *inside yourself* to become a Naturopath. The challenges you take on to your heart, mind and soul when you decide to take on the authority to heal. Believe me, compared to that, the schoolin' is the easy part.

First, I want to be sure to clarify the difference between a "correspondence school" and an "online degree". I myself received my initial valuable education through an approved correspondence school. Detractors of Traditional Naturopathy are quick to "caution" people that many Naturopaths get their degrees "online", as if prestigious institutions from Harvard University to the University of Phoenix and a jillion others are not likewise offering correspondence education these days! Truth is, the world is a much different place than it used to be, and more and more aspects of our lives are occurring "online". *Where you were sitting* while you were learning seems to be of great concern to the AANP licensing advocates. For us, the traditional group, we're far more concerned with the content of *what* we are learning than *where* we are sitting when that learning occurs.

In Traditional Naturopathy approved schools we study the properties of herbs, the functions of vitamins and minerals in the body, nutrition, chemistry, homeopathy, anatomy and physiology, the properties of massage and reflexology, and in my case (although not in all schools), about Bach Flower remedies and how to actually make your own herbal teas, tinctures, salves and pills (all of which I had to turn in to be graded). We also get a few basic business classes, write book reports and listen to lectures on various conditions and global health problems. We listen to the instructors lecture, read and write reports, sit for proctored exams and receive our grades. Wow, sounds a lot like...school... doesn't it? That's because that's what it is – school! Not some diploma mill that churns out degrees to any creep with a hundred bucks. An approved *school*. Readin' writin' and 'rithmatic.

Think about it. At a traditional university or college you usually follow this pattern: You get up in the morning, go to your classes, listen to lectures, then you go home with homework to complete and turn in. When it's time, you take proctored exams to test your knowledge, you're graded on your comprehension, and you can't advance unless you pass. Well, that's the same thing many of us do without sitting in a classroom.

For the many *many* of us (like me) who are working at jobs while we go to school, it goes more like this: You come home from work, eat dinner, listen to lectures on tape or by Internet, then complete and turn in your homework. When it's time, you take proctored exams to test your knowledge, you're graded on your comprehension, and you can't advance unless you pass. Hmm. Pretty darn close isn't it? Speaking for myself, I worked a full-time job all day then came home and spent nearly every night and entire weekends studying my butt off!

It's plain to see that a correspondence school can very easily give the same level of education that you would get in a more *conventional* school, with the added bonus being that we have to show that we have enough commitment to our course of study to keep doing it with no one watching over our shoulders to make sure we make it to class! In the traditional approved schools, you can get a very good grounding and education in *Traditional* Naturopathy studying by correspondence. Notice I stressed "traditional" because the things we *don't* study in our correspondence courses that the AANP schools do, are courses such as how to take x-rays, how to prescribe prescription drugs, gynecological rotations and how to do stitches and other minor surgical procedures. If I wanted to do those kinds of things, I'd have gone to Allopathic medical school and become an MD. So being that I'm a Naturopath, I took Naturopathic courses. Enough said.

During an industry convention, a person who was just starting out asked me what was the hardest part of my first year in practice. After much thought I replied "Learning how to talk to people about their bowel movements with a straight face." I don't think this was what she was expecting to hear, but to a large degree it's the truth. After all, this is not something we are used to doing, yet it is vital to a person's health. Although they might exist, I've never met anyone at a cocktail party who just said out of nowhere, "You know, I usually have two bowel movements a day, but I find that it is very dependant on how much water I drink. So how about those Knicks?" I mean, face it. If someone did say that to *you*, you'd probably find something else to do, quickly. And yet it is just these mundane aspects that often make up "the hard part".

Often I have asked myself how crazy a person needs to be to do this. This may give you some idea, or at least how it happened for me:

First; you make a decision that you're the kind of person who can take the authority to heal, although it's probably a good thing you don't know what this really means before you take this on. You think you do, but you don't.

Second; you pick a school and go there. This step is what I refer to (believe it or not) as "the easy part". Again, you don't think so while you're doing it, but that's how it turns out.

Third; you go into practice. This is scary. It takes a certain amount of trust and guts to just hang out a shingle and hope that the clients will come. In addition to all the mental/emotional/ what-have-I-done vortex, I will tell you that once I got my office opened, the phones turned on, and the fax, copier, etc. purchased, I had $126.00 left in my bank account. Good thing my landlord didn't know that. Luckily for her (and me) my ball got rolling very quickly and it has continued to roll ever since.

Fourth; you take on anyone with anything that comes in. Since we see the body as a whole (most Naturopaths don't specialize), you have to be willing to tackle anything that comes through the door. This can get pretty bizarre at times. As I've said, my comfortable notion that as a Naturopath I would mostly be giving nutritional, exercise and supplement advice to primarily healthy people got quickly shattered and I found myself immersed almost immediately into a world of "throw-aways". Throw-aways are all the people who have been told by other doctors that they either can't be helped so "just get used to" their problem, or have been told to "Go home and get your affairs in order."

Now *there* is a scary phrase for you, "Get your affairs in order." A friend of mine jokingly says that I should combine my practice with a health spa and call it "The Last Resort", since we get told that we are just that by so many people. It always seems odd to me when someone tells me that, "You're my last resort." Before what exactly? You know what? On second thought, don't tell me. I think the statement alone is sufficient pressure. Thanks.

You also need to actively listen to and accept what people say to you. It is not my place to judge; it is my place to listen and be respectful. Not that I won't call someone on an out-and-out lie, such as telling me that he's been taking a supplement very religiously when I know for a fact that he didn't have enough to last them a month and didn't purchase more, but for the most part I try not to make judgment calls.

For example I once had a lady come in who, despite the fact that she was on five different prescription blood pressure medications, still had BP levels that were staying in the 200-something-over-150ish range, which is stroke territory. When I asked her opinion as to why this might have been happening, she exchanged a meaningful glance and nod with her husband and then told me that she had had a UFO experience. Apparently she'd been fine until a UFO had hovered over and stopped her car, and all of a sudden, from that moment on, her blood pressure had gone crazy. Her sister, who had been in the car with her, had already experienced a stroke and had died. So okay.

All I know is that when we got her radiation lowered using homeopathy and detox, her doctor actually took her off all her prescriptions and she regained her health. I don't have to know *why* it happened, it just did! She was very grateful that I accepted the UFO story at face value, but why wouldn't I? I wasn't there, so who am I to judge? And believe it or not, this was not the oddest story I've been told by a client. Far from it as a matter of fact. By the way, an interesting side note to this story is that the lady I just described lives very near Roswell, New Mexico.

But after these tasks are established, you suddenly find yourself in a conundrum. How will people know what I do if I can't tell them? The ever-changing laws on natural medicine are very restrictive. Not only can we not "diagnose, treat or cure" anything, we're not allowed to discuss our track record either. If someone asks what my success rate is with, let's say, cancer, I can't tell them. I am allowed to discuss failures (thanks so much), just not successes. This leaves me with very little to talk about.

You take a profession where most people only have a hazy idea of what we do in the first place, and then we're not allowed to tell them! The upside is that if I ever decide to change professions I could probably be a very good politician. I can now talk for an hour without committing to anything; something I couldn't do before. Everything gets couched with legally-correct-mumbo-jumbo and mumbling about "improving the immune system" and "stress reduction".

Though truthfully, improving immune system function and reducing stress in the body are in fact what Naturopaths do. We're just not allowed to say *how*, or what we hope the outcome will be, or how it has been for others in the past. You think you have it rough! Try being effective with both your hands and your tongue tied behind your back sometime. And yet, effective we still are. Naturopaths around the country still manage to be effective and heal under these ridiculous circumstances. God bless us, every one. And bless doubly the clients who trustingly place their lives in our shackled but well-meaning hands.

It is this very same political hokey-pokey that I am discussing here that causes the biggest problem for a lot of Naturopaths. In an attempt to stay under the radar of law makers (and trouble makers), some find themselves so tongue-tied that they become ineffective, and being the good people that most Naturopaths are (okay, I'm prejudiced), they quit when they feel they are no longer effective. The burn-out rate for Naturopaths is exceedingly high, and I think this hog-tying is a lot more responsible for this issue than anything else. It turns caring, educated and responsible healers into tongue-tied, frustrated, teeth-grinding crazy people. I am far from the only Naturopath who has TMJ from clenching my teeth all day! I'd call it more of an "occupational hazard" for us. It gets very frustrating for the clients sometimes as well, but if you don't like how we have to talk to you, contact your Congressman. It isn't our first choice either, and we can't do a thing about it.

The hardest part of my second year in practice was learning that you can lead a horse to water, but you can't make it take its supplements. At first, when clients did not adhere to the protocols I outlined for them, I blamed myself – I must not have been convincing enough, I wasn't clear enough about it, I didn't stress the importance enough, and on and on. Near the end of my second year I realized that you just can't reach everyone. That sounds simple, but it wasn't for me.

Later down the line I watched an associate I was training who was a few years behind me, go through the same thing: "Maybe if I'd just said this..." and on and on. I hoped that he would learn, but he didn't. He let it burn him out instead. That may sound kind of tough, but that's the way it is. No matter how well you express yourself, no matter how deep your knowledge and commitment are, you just can't *get* through to some people. And then there is attachment to illness, which was a real shocker for me. That is discussed more in depth in another chapter, so I'll let it go here for now.

If this next part sounds at all immodest, then so be it – it needs to be said. It takes an enormous amount of courage to do this job, in many different ways. For instance, it takes a good dose of chutzpah for a 5'5", 115-pound woman to look a 240-pound football coach in the eye and tell him he can't eat bread and white potatoes anymore! And even more to get him to do it! By the way, he's no longer 240 pounds, but he can still be very intimidating nonetheless. When I see him at the health food store, he waves cheerily and says "Hi! I hate you." He's still mad at me about the bread and potatoes, but his body isn't, so I can live with that.

Keeping the Courage

It takes a lot of guts to know every day that you can be harassed, arrested and/or jailed just for saying a wrong word, or even because you've been quoted wrongly by someone else. Yet you keep going. Day after day, year after year, because you believe in what you're doing. And having the knowledge that if someone really wants to get you, they will. A few years ago a Naturopath in Minnesota told a planted investigator doing his best to entrap her that she thought he may have some back problems, and might want to see a chiropractor. Based on this, she was accused of "diagnosing" a back problem (he had said it hurt) and her practice was shut down while she was "investigated".

One of the tough aspects of the job for me is that it takes a lot of courage to keep taking on the throw-aways, which is what Naturopaths do. To be able to say, "Okay, let's get the facts straight. You're in Stage 4 cancer, you've had chemo, surgery and radiation, you're missing a few vital organs and your doctor has told you that there is no point in doing anything more, and to go home and 'get your affairs in order,' is that correct? Okay, well, we better get started and see what we can do", and mean it. This is far from the only thing we deal with, but it happens often enough. Even one takes a lot of courage, and it doesn't get any easier. I never have gotten used to it. It takes the most courage (the most from your soul) to be able to spend your life every day looking at carnage and not give up. Not on them, and not on your practice.

It all gets so frustrating at times. I couldn't begin to count how many people have come in as human train wrecks, so I fix them up, and then they go out and do the same thing over again. And over, and over. Sometimes their particular loaded gun is food or lifestyle choices, but maybe the most frustrating is their doctors. It's amazing how many times I have cleaned up the side effects of medications, then the folks go right back to the firing line again. Part of this, of course, is because we were not allowed by law to be as clear as we might have wanted to be that the condition they had was *caused* by drug side effects in the first place, but even some of the ones who understand this will still go back for more of the same.

And the worst part, the excuse we hear most often is, "My insurance covers the doctor, but it won't cover you." Great. You only had to pay a $20 co-pay to get this rash, or joint pain or nausea or whatever you are currently experiencing. And have you forgotten how much you pay per month for your insurance? So they come to me again, and I fix them up, again, until the next time. And you just keep thinking, why, why, why? Why would you do this to yourself? But that's the kind of thinking that gets Naturopaths in trouble. We can't tell them to not take their prescriptions or to quit damaging themselves, so we refer to information in books and websites and just keep fixing them up again. If I have one more person say, "Gee, I get this huge rash every time I take antibiotics. Weird, huh?" Then they keep taking them! It's sort of like, "Gee, it hurts every time I hit myself with this hammer. Weird, huh?" Not really.

Another frustrating thing to deal with: People lie. They do this for a variety of reasons, but it's undeniably and clearly detrimental to their process. For example, if I'm working with someone regarding Candida and we just can't seem to get rid of it, I say, "Are you taking your supplements? Are you avoiding sugar, alcohol and breads?" and she says, "Yes, Shauna." I have a tendency to believe this. So I start changing around what they're taking, coming up with new strategies, all kinds of things, when in fact, I'm really not helping. I'm resorting to Plan B, when they haven't even tried Plan A properly! After a while, I just have to do the math. Look at what they've purchased against what I've suggested. Then we have to have "The Talk". That's where I ask them if they're really serious about their health or not. And the thing is, *I* hate "The Talk" only slightly less than *they* hate "The Talk". I'd much rather just have someone admit, "Man I blew it", and then get back on track, than to run both of us in circles. This wastes a lot of time all around.

However, sometimes people lie simply because something is just too embarrassing to talk about. This kind of lying I can better understand, and am therefore more tolerant of it, but it still doesn't help. I had a client, a nice guy from Alabama, with whom I went around and around looking for the source of his problem. Even though it was embarrassing for him, it helped enormously when he finally came clean and told me that just prior to his unexplained symptoms kicking in, he and his buddies had gotten drunk on a camping trip and eaten a half-cooked raccoon. Aha! Got it now.

It is also a mystery to me as to why people are fine with taking handfuls of prescription drugs, but consider supplements as "so inconvenient". What? Why? Don't you just line them up and swallow them just like other pills? That's how I take mine. Yes, admittedly there are practitioners out there who ramp people up too much, asking them to take huge amounts of supplements multiple times a day, but as mentioned earlier, I'm not one of those practitioners. I try to keep people on the minimum of what they need, and then they can decide if they want more supplements to optimize the effect. *Note to any Naturopaths reading this: This is a very effective way of suggesting supplements. According to others in the field, my rate of compliance among clients is much better than average.*

Think for a moment about all the things you do everyday for your safety that are inconvenient. It would be a lot easier to not lock, and therefore have to unlock, our cars and houses multiple times a day, but we do it for our security. We look both ways before crossing the street. We cook and store our food in ways that avoid contamination and spoilage. Wouldn't be a lot easier to just leave that chicken out on the counter before you cook it? Sure it would. But the consequences...yuck.

My Love Affair with Water

Okay, I know you're going to think I'm kidding on this one, but it's totally true. One of the hardest things I do is to get people to drink enough water! I could say to many people that they needed to eat kitty litter, and they would say "The kind with the scent crystals, or..?", but man, don't ask them to drink more water! The longer I'm in practice and the more I continue my self-education, the more I realize and appreciate that water is the gift of life and health. I would provide incomplete sessions with my clients if I did not emphasize this perfect substance.

Now before you go all judgmental on me, ask yourself, are you drinking enough water? And by enough I mean half your pounds of body weight in ounces each and every day – If you are a 150-pound person, are you drinking 75 ounces of water every day? Gotcha, didn't I? There went your comfortable notion of "Oh I drink lots of water", the line that I hear dozens of times a week from dehydrated people. However, you're not alone. According to studies, about 75% of Americans are *chronically* dehydrated, a fact confirmed not only by teams of experts, but by my receptionist Judy, who is a wonderful massage therapist. While working on me one day, she commented that it was nice to work on someone who is hydrated, so I asked her what percentage of her clients did she feel were hydrated. She thought for a long moment then said "Well, there's you...". Wow, sad.

It's amazing how many of the most common complaints I hear from people can be connected to dehydration. Constipation, headaches, fatigue, weight problems, lack of focus, joint and back pain and hunger pangs to name just a few. I remember a college student who came in after seeing multiple doctors and neurologists and still had chronic migraines. The pain pills she was prescribed did a good job at curing consciousness, but her headaches were still with her. When asked, she told me that due to her busy schedule of classes and work, she was only drinking two or three glasses of water a day. She started drinking seven (correct amount for her body weight) and the chronic headaches went away, bada-bing, just like that in a matter of weeks.

According to the same study quoted above, even a 2% drop in hydration is capable of triggering problems in short-term memory, fatigue (lack of water being the number one trigger in daytime fatigue), and will slow metabolism. Joint and back pain was reduced in about 80% of sufferers tested. And one University of Washington study showed that drinking water also cut down late night hunger pangs in nearly 100% of dieters in their study. Not terribly good news for Haagen-Dazs®, but good news for you! Still not convinced? How about this: Being sufficiently hydrated has been shown to cause a significant drop in cancer risk. Yes, *cancer*. Colon cancer by 45%, bladder cancer by 50%, and a walloping 79% drop in breast cancer. Just by drinking water!

My secret for drinking all the water you need is simple: Small doses of room temperature water throughout the day. If you drink a big glass of water all at once, true, you'll flush most of it about 15 minutes later. My advice for clients is to get a big glass (mine's purple and sits on my desk at all times) or a marked container and fill it with the water you need to drink over the day. Then drink it a swallow or two at a time, throughout the day. One friend of mine trained himself on one of his frequent long drives. I told him to just take a sip of water at the start of every third song he heard on the radio. He drank two liters of water and ran out of gas before he needed a pit stop. Not rocket science is it? But if you do it every day, it will keep you hydrated. Enough said.

Occupational Hazards

After you've been in practice a while and you have clients coming from all around the country (or the world in our case) another difficult thing rears its head: Living up to your own reputation. Once you rack up a certain amount of success stories, including some pretty dramatic ones, people start to have some mighty high expectations. One woman came in with Stage 4 cancer (not that unusual), but she had also had *eight* internal organs removed by surgery including part of her liver, a kidney and a lung. I explained to her that as a Naturopath, the only thing I could do was try to get her body functioning normally again. So with eight organs missing, how close to "normal" did she really think we could come?

Truth is, she wasn't really thinking, she was just desperate. People also have a tendency to forget that you only get out of it what you put into it. While it is true that some clients' friends/siblings/bosses/whomevers had faster progress than they might be experiencing, they also need to bear in mind that the person who referred them was surely doing what was called for: Supplements, exercise, proper diet and water. Sitting on the couch eating chips and only taking your supplements sporadically will never work out well. And some conditions just flat take longer to respond. Let me be clear about this: I do not have a magic bullet or a magic wand, and I do not think such a thing exists. And even if it did, how would I even charge for using it?

At the onset of my practice, a weird thing I never before considered that I now live with regularly is that it takes a certain constitution to just go about your life without losing your mind due to the variety of knowledge you accrue. As one example, when taking my turn on an elliptical machine at the local Rec Center, I grasped the padded handles and squeezed a copious quantity of heaven knows how many other people's sweat down onto my wrists. The Latin names for all the various bacteria associated with such an action immediately sprang into my head, making me immediately slightly nauseous (I mean, where have those palms *been*? Sorry if you've just eaten). I felt better after I washed my hands for a long time and resolved to buy a pair of workout gloves, but the knowledge itself had already made me queasy. Similarly, a friend of mine in California once had a not-so-minor flip-out over dust mites, something most people might never have heard of, but that he had intimate (and microscopic) knowledge of.

A really annoying aspect of my career is that I'm also now nearly impossible to watch TV with, since the sheer number of drug ads with their insane disclosure warnings will drive me bonkers long before the desired one-hour episode of "Dances with the Stars" has ended. I can easily launch into detailed lists of absurdities with many of these popular and ubiquitous commercials, but I shall just present one here as I'm trying to contain myself.

While trying to watch a movie at home one night, a drug ad for a commonly prescribed asthma inhaler came on. Even though I was paying very little attention to it (the teeth clenching thing again), a phrase stated very quickly and kind of slurred caught my attention. I sat straight up thinking, "Did I hear what I think I just heard?" Surely not. So I kept watching, knowing they'd probably repeat the commercial later. They did, I paid careful attention this time. Sure enough, in the middle of the commercial the voiceover said that this drug "wasn't for everyone" since it increased the incidence of "asthma-related death". *WHAT?* Death? If it increases the risk of asthma-related death, should it be for *anyone*? So I went to the PDR website, and there it was: "Increased incidence of asthma-related death" as a listed, and *acceptable*, side effect. For an asthma medication. And people still take it in droves. This scares me and makes me want to go ballistic at the same time. It's really hard to not let this type of thing get you down.

When it does, a friend of mine (a woman whose humor is as dark as mine) gets my sense of humor kick-started again with an adage like, "It's nothing a bottle of Jack and a bell tower won't solve." Sometimes, all you can do is laugh. Either that or go crazy. It's just that it can be such an uphill battle.

I admit to having a hard time holding my tongue and not looking like either a know-it-all or a freak with strangers. I have often stood in the grocery store while someone shopping with their children in front of me unloads their cart full of powdered drink mixes loaded with artificial sweeteners and other toxins, hot dogs, potato chips, sodas and diet sodas, lunch meats full of nitrates and MSG – in general a cart full of poison. What I'd love to say at times is, "Are you *trying* to cause ADHD and/or kill your children?" But of course you run the risk of someone calling the cops. So instead I hum and think about baseball. One simple note for the grocery store: If you can't pronounce the ingredients on a label, or a food is blue, don't eat it. There are no blue foods in nature. And for those of you who just said,"Uh, Shauna, what about blueberries?", shame on you. If you look at them, blueberries are actually *purple*, not blue.

As much as I am trying to keep this light, I must cop to a not-so-humorous aspect of this concept. I will admit to a "dark night of the soul" situation I had to learn to accept and overcome a few years into practice. It started with the dreams. The worst of them was one where I was standing in a large warehouse watching live people go by on conveyor belts. As they went by, people in scrubs and surgical masks would either cut into these people pulling something out of them then stuffing it back in before they went by on the belt, or would inject them (mostly the babies) with something that would cause parts of them to shrivel and die off or to go into seizures.

Another one involved very sick and dying people who were standing in line. They would walk up to me, one by one, and we'd talk about what was wrong with them. Then they'd thank me and move on. After this went on for awhile, I'd think, "Man! How many of these people are there?" I walked around the corner and saw that this line of sick people extended far into the horizon; it seemed never ending. These were not good dreams, and it was not a good time in my life. This, I believe is known as "internalizing". Whatever it's called, it sucked.

And as if your own mind wasn't impishly bad enough, there is the more serious outside persecution. Just when you think the Salem trials are dead, here they come again. This is a time-honored tradition among great thinkers and healers, so I try to think of it as a badge of honor. After all, am I not following in the great footsteps of Harold Hoxey, Rene Caisse and Hulda Clark? Or at least that's the story I tell myself. I met a man (in a program designed to help people better handle stress incidentally) who told me that poor Hulda Clark ended up having to be escorted out of her clinic at night (accompanied by him and two others) wearing body armor! Gee, do you think Christian Barnard had these kinds of problems? I think not.

Anyway, some of this outright persecution comes from the usual suspects: Allopathic doctors, their close-knit buddies in the pharmaceutical industry, local jealousy, but as much as I hate to say it, a lot of it comes from other Naturopaths on either side of the Traditional Naturopath/Naturopathic Physician issue (see the chapter Naturopath vs. Naturopath). The worst, though not the only harassment I've endured has been from a local "Physician-style" Naturopath. She has some very strong opinions that she voices whenever she feels the whim in the local paper or to whomever will listen. The newspaper seems to love her for some reason. Every time she has an "opinion" it gets printed. I, on the other hand, won an international scientific award (twice), and the paper's editor said he "didn't have enough room to print it." Ever. Oh well, I'm sure the locals were enriched by the recipes for "Fresh Summer Salads" that they did have the room to print.

Mostly the stuff I get from her and her group are garden variety nuisance tactics–threatening phone calls and letters, coming to my public seminars and being disruptive, notes on my car, etc. Someone got stuck on the word "crucify" for a while ("We're going to crucify you") and I wasn't sure whether to be concerned or complimented. Finally I settled on apathy. FYI to those folks: A death threat scrawled on a powder-pink Post-it® is *not* having the desired scary effect. In fact, I'd like to thank whoever did that one because that was when I lost my concern and started laughing at all this nonsense.

Once a group of these AANP-types (by coincidence there are a number of them in my town, lucky me) got together and came as a group (mob) to one of my seminars in a bold attempt to disrupt it. Unfortunately for them, I was away at a training seminar and my associate was giving the lecture that night. Secure in the knowledge of his topic, he held his own very well against the whole group, and in fact they made themselves look pretty foolish to other attendees. So they contented themselves with issuing him dark and dire warnings about me, and suggesting that they would hire him. Man! Disrupting a seminar *and* trying to steal my employees? I ask you: Is this any way for professionals to act?

Although I don't pretend to understand the animosity directed at me from some fellow Naturopaths, I do understand why the pharmaceutical industry is against all of us as a whole. Once in the shower, where I do my best thinking, I pondered how much money the natural medicine industry is actually costing the pharmaceutical industry. When I went into work that day I grabbed a client chart at random. This particular client had been on three prescriptions that she was supposed to stay on for the rest of her life, if not for her doctor taking her off them because we were able to eliminate her symptoms.

I took the generic cost of those three meds and totaled up what they cost her per month. Then I multiplied that by how many months she would be around and not taking them (I used age 78, as that is what insurance companies use as the average mortality rate). It came to around $300,000.00 just for that one person! Our practice and many others have clients numbering in the thousands. That should give you a good idea on what they have against us. We are very bad for their business – and proud of it I might add. So I guess if you run into persecution, hold your head high and try like the dickens to find a way to laugh about it.

And here's one more thing they'll never tell you in school. This job is really tough on personal relationships. For one thing, as hard as I try not to be "preachy" or "judgmental" it's awfully hard to watch people you care about do dumb things that are so bad for them without commenting. I once had to break up with a perfectly nice guy because of his diet soda habit. I just couldn't watch him drink ant poison! Another definition of a "drinking problem" I guess.

And then there's the fact that after looking at carnage all day long it's rough sometimes to get in a jolly mood when you go home. As hard as I try, it's difficult at times to go home and spin plates or balance balls on my nose. Some days are just flat hard to take, and I doubt I'm much fun after them. While it's one thing to intellectually understand that working with sick people is challenging work, it's another thing altogether to have someone crying and begging you to help them while sitting in your office.

If you're going to do this, just go into it with the knowledge that you have to surround yourself with very understanding people, or you may have to go it alone. Fortunately now I have someone who sends me off to work by saying "Work hard. Heal everyone." He gets me, but that hasn't always been the case. It's an amazing, wonderful, incredible gift to heal for a living, and there's nothing else I would rather do. But it's not always easy.

So what does it take to be a Naturopath? Mostly a lot of study with an open and inquisitive mind, an earnest desire to help, massive determination, a caring heart, a weird sense of humor, and one very sturdy suit of armor.

CHAPTER 6

"Dis-eases"

"Drugs never cure disease. They merely hush the voice of nature's protest, and pull down the danger signals she erects along the pathway of transgression. Any poison taken into the system has to be reckoned with later even though it palliates present symptoms. Pain may disappear, but the patient is left in worse condition, though unconscious of it at the time."

— Daniel H. Kress, M.D.

Okay, here it is, right off the bat. One of those massive, general sweeping statements that everyone keeps telling me I'm going to get in trouble for making, but here goes. I don't even *believe* in many named "diseases", such as cancer, Lupus, Fibromyalgia or many others. In fact most Naturopaths don't even refer to "disease" but rather "dis-*ease*" meaning that there is an imbalance, or a lack of ease in the body. And I *really* don't believe in "auto-immune" diseases. Since Naturopaths are not allowed to diagnose, this is probably a good thing. However since I realize that making this statement will cause many to think I'm an idiot, let me explain what I mean.

Chickenpox: Now that's my idea of a disease. You catch the Varicella virus for the first time and you get Chickenpox. End of story. A specific virus that causes a specific condition and set of symptoms. Most "diseases" now days are not like that. Most of them are merely a group of symptoms that get *classified* as being a certain disease. At a seminar I was teaching, a woman asked me what the difference was between Chronic Fatigue Syndrome,

Epstein-Barr and Fibromyalgia. I gave her a list of symptoms; fatigue, pain, and depression, then asked her to give them back to me in any order. She said, "Pain, fatigue, depression." I said, "Fibromyalgia." She said, "Fatigue, pain, depression." I said, "Chronic Fatigue." She said, "Depression, pain, fatigue." I said, "Epstein-Barr." You get the point. Same stuff, different order. It's all the same to me whatever you name it. Potato, po*tah*to.

Now to address "auto-immunity". Hmm. The very idea of a person's immune system getting so strong that the body "attacks itself" just seems whack to me. How can your immune system be *too* strong so that it over-reacts? Immune systems are meant to be strong! Rheumatoid Arthritis, Bird Flu, Lupus, a lot of conditions fall into this category. My theory is that the *reverse* is actually true. Let me give you the analogy I use in seminars: Let's say that you're home alone at night. You're in the kitchen and suddenly you hear a loud noise out in the yard. Between you and the yard is a big, bolted, secure door. You look out the window, maybe turn on a light out there, if it's really extreme you may even call the cops to check it out. The point is, you'll react reasonably because you know you're safe behind that strong locked door. You forget about it and go on with your night.

Second scenario: You're home alone at night. You're in the kitchen and suddenly you hear a loud noise out in the yard. Between you and the unknown source of noise in the yard is a flimsy, rickety screen door that a toddler could stick his arm through. So do you react in the same manner? No way! First you yelp and jump half out of your skin, then start tearing around looking for something to defend yourself with – a baseball bat, a gun, some artificial sweetener, whatever potentially deadly thing you can find. Instead of the aloof "Hey, what was that?" reaction you had when you were behind a securely locked door, you had the freaked out "What the F&#*! was that?" and "Get me outta' here" reaction. And then you lay awake all night wondering if whatever made that noise is still hanging around.

So while it is true that inflammation is an over-reaction, in my mind it's not because your defenses were too strong, but rather because they were so weak. Ah so – You're getting it now, aren't you Grasshopper? Are you seeing my point?

How about cancer? Well, you don't *catch* cancer! No one sneezes on you and you get cancer. Cancer is a group of mutated cells that got out of hand, like a mob riot. So the question is; what caused those cells to mutate in the first place? In my mind, what the person "has", if we must classify it, is whatever caused the cell mutation to occur. The group of symptoms may be called "cancer", but if you want to stop it and keep it from coming back, you'll need to figure out what caused it. I don't see people with "cancer" so much as I see people with various types of poisoning that have caused a growth and/or mutation to occur.

Something else you virtually never hear: Cancer is one of the most avoidable "dis-eases" out there. With the billions and billions of dollars raised for cancer "research", when was the last time you heard one of these oh-so-benevolent cancer societies mention that you can *avoid* cancer in the first place mostly with food, water and lifestyle choices? To reiterate an earlier point: According to many studies, 75% of Americans are chronically dehydrated. Do you think that people in general might be encouraged to drink more water if one of the big cancer societies mentioned that being sufficiently hydrated cuts your risk of colon cancer by 45%, bladder cancer by 50%, and breast cancer by 79%? How fast would people run for a new "vaccine" or pill that could make the claim of preventing cancers by even a measly 10-20%??

Or do you think that if they told people that their microwave oven was turning grains, meats, milk, and both frozen and raw fruits and vegetables into indigestible carcinogens and have been found to be a cause behind tumors and growths in the stomach and intestines, people might cut down their usage of them? Or, heaven forbid, demand that restaurants not use them? There are *big* dollars being raised for cancer research and treatment, so why is there virtually none being spent on educating the public as to what they can do to avoid it all together? *Because there is no profit in avoiding cancer.* Bleak, but true.

And let's talk about "depression" as a disease. First of all, you need to realize that in order to prescribe a pill for a condition, it needs to be classified as a disease. This is why conditions like depression, obesity and alcoholism are all now being referred to as "diseases". And don't even get me started on "diseases" like Restless Leg Syndrome! In my experience, the feeling of being depressed is often just a sounding smoke alarm of sorts, a warning that something else is wrong in the body – Panic attacks particularly. If something is amiss, your body will get upset about it, hence, depression or panic. Often when you clear up the imbalance the "depression" just goes away on its own, like smoke drifting out of a room.

There is a HUGE market for anti-depressants, easily some of the most commonly prescribed drugs, and it's sickening to me how many young children and teenagers are now taking them. No one wants to feel lousy all the time, so they're in great demand. What I think what mostly they represent are band-aids that covers up deeper issues. Realize here that I'm not talking about situational depression. That of course, is a different story. A loved one dies, you get a divorce, your partner is chronically ill, whatever. But my opinion is that even situational depression is better handled than covered up. I'm a big fan of talk therapy in these situations; with a pastor or a therapist or someone else trained in these areas preferably, but even with a friend if the situation is not too dire. What I want to address here though, is depression with no apparent cause. Notice I said "apparent" because to me, everything has a cause.

Let's review at a few scenarios here again: You're told that you're about to die or even to be sick for the rest of your life. In any normal human being, this will cause depression. If it doesn't, there may be something else wrong with you! So if something is going on that you may not be aware of, but your body is, *it's* going to get depressed, therefore *you* feel depressed. Instead of taking a pill that covers the alarm going off, it may behoove you to try to figure out what might be bugging your body.

Next, if you fall into the water and start choking and can't breathe, what's going to happen? You're going to panic. This is your body's way of saying "Hello! I can't breathe. Need a little help here!" So if you're experiencing *panic attacks*, there's a very good chance that something is cutting off your air, water or nutritional supply. Get the supply line back, panic stops. Just makes so much sense, doesn't it? Therein you find one of the basics of natural medicine: It makes sense. And as Judge Judy always says from the bench, "If it doesn't make sense, it's probably wrong."

Arthritis is an interesting catch-all phrase for all kinds of pain. How can you have arthritis in say, one finger? If your immune system is making the body "attack itself", then why would it only attack a finger or a toe and not your whole body? I once saw a woman who was on a very serious drug that suppresses your immune system with *very* severe side effects (just the TV commercial warnings will keep you up nights) because her right hand pinkie knuckle hurt, mostly when she played tennis. Many times this is the sort of damage that may be able to be cleared up by a chiropractor, osteopath or even supplements, but instead she was prescribed a drug that gave her an increased risk of infections, TB, and all kinds of other horrendous side-effects.

The important thing to remember is that the condition called "arthritis" can have many different causes. And a good rule of thumb is if your pain pill for arthritis isn't working, *you probably don't have arthritis*, and it may be time to start looking for other answers. One good thing you can say about pain pills, they work! My joint pain in the months when I had Lyme Disease was described as "arthritic" but in fact was just a side effect of my Lyme's, so it left when the bacteria left. So was that arthritis, or Lyme Disease? I can't even begin to figure out how many people within my practice have had their arthritis symptoms disappear when they were simply detoxed from Candida. So was it arthritis, or Candida? Answer: Who cares? As long as you get out of your pain, who cares about what it was labeled?

Among the myriad of issues I have found that cause or contribute to "arthritis" symptoms include: Candida, parasites, synovial fluid toxicity and/or inflammation (usually from flu shots or other vaccines), various viruses or bacteria, dehydration, and lack of fatty acids. Even the "osteo" type of arthritis had to have had a cause in the first place, and if you can get that cleared up, then the cartilage has a shot at healthier regeneration. Many people have now recognized the benefits of gluocosamine-chondroitin in that process.

Similarly, what is the "diagnosis" of Rheumatoid Arthritis all about? Pain and inflammation in the joints, sometimes with degeneration. Now, what is causing the inflammation? Hmm. See? No wonder we Naturopaths don't need to diagnose.

The Lyme Disease Conundrum

Getting back to Lyme Disease: Number one, it's very tricky. A lot of people have now heard of Lyme Disease, and they've usually taken away that it's caused by tick bites. Well, yes and no. Lyme Disease can be caused by a tick bite (as with my own experience), but there are a number of other ways to contract it. As a matter of fact, a research facility in Nevada that does very little else but research Lyme Disease estimates that about 85% of Americans have the Lyme bacterial spirochete (*Borrelia burgdorferi* in case you're interested) in their bloodstream. So based on their research they're now thinking that you don't need to have a tick bite you to get it, and instead it can be passed from person to person in about the same easy ways as Hepatitis B – that is saliva, blood and bodily fluid contact. So if a restaurant waiter has it and doesn't wash his hands between his trip to the men's room and serving your food, you could get it. That easy.

Someone could sneeze on you and you're not aware of it, or you could get exposed by picking up a piece of produce in the grocery store that somebody just had their bacteria-laden fingers on. Just another good reason to make a 500-pound-gorilla out of your immune system – you just never know when you're going to get exposed to something. No, I'm *not* trying to turn you into a germophobe, just trying to get across the point of how important it is to keep your immune system healthy!

Anyway, Lyme's is one of those things that mimics many other diseases, including but not limited to rheumatoid arthritis,

Epstein-Barr, Fibromyalgia, Chronic Fatigue and a lot of these "new" diseases floating around. Think about it for a moment. Remember the 1970's (if you can). Had you ever even heard the word "Fibromyalgia"? Me neither. Now, how many people that you currently know have been handed that diagnosis? If you leave your house at all, chances are you know quite a few. For me, I don't think a day goes by that I'm not working with someone who tells me he or she has been diagnosed with Fibromyalgia.

Another problem with Lyme Disease (though it's not exclusive to Lyme's) is that people will manifest symptoms very differently. Some are hit quicker than others (mine was nearly instantaneous) while others go on for quite a while with "flu-like" symptoms that come and go before anything more severe pops up. And since the Lyme's bacteria is classified as a "stealth virus" (meaning a virus that actually penetrates inside your cells and/ or DNA as opposed to hanging out on the outside of a cell like a regular virus), it can hide out in your system for a very long time then rear its ugly head when your immune system is suppressed from stress and/or a minor virus.

This is one of the reasons that it's a real bugger for a doctor to diagnose. If you get a tick bite that you're aware of and a few hours or a few days later you have a raging fever, sore throat, vicious headache, joint pain and a bulls-eye rash around the bite as I did, then it's a slam dunk. Most cases are not that clear cut. For one thing, you may not even know you got a tick bite in the first place. Ticks like out-of-the-way places so very often people are bitten on the head where their hair obscures the rash, or in an armpit or other relatively unseen spot. Not everyone gets it right in the middle of the belly as I did (I looked like an archery target), or even gets the classic "bulls-eye" rash. Sometimes it's just reddish or blotchy like from poison ivy or a garden variety insect bite.

As you can tell from the description above, this is a very painful condition. Most people when faced with horrible headaches and body pain will immediately reach for anti-inflammatories like Motrin®, Advil® or Tylenol®, and this is yet another of the problems with the diagnosis process. If you have been taking an

NSAID or other anti-inflammatory, the blood marker for Lyme's has a very good chance of not showing up at all. Something about the anti-inflammatory can make it disappear. So even if you do get a blood test, it may not be completely accurate. Then if you are diagnosed with it, often there isn't a whole lot that can be done anyway.

The usual protocol for Lyme Disease is daily massive doses of antibiotics, many of which the Lyme's bacteria seems to have already figured a way around. Bacteria and viruses are like cockroaches in that way, in that they always seem to figure out how to survive, and Lyme Disease has passed into the large and ever-growing spectrum of diseases that are primarily "antibiotic resistant". One woman I saw with Lyme Disease was a miserable walking skeleton – not from the disease mind you, but from over five years of taking 1,500 mg of strong antibiotics every day.

So how do Naturopaths work with a dis-ease such as Lyme's? Here's a seemingly simplistic answer from a Chinatown "pharmacist" (he's actually a doctor in China) that I knew in the 1980's in Los Angeles. I was having a conversation with him as to what he knew about what was still being called the "Gay Plague" at the time as the labels HIV and AIDS hadn't been coined yet.

He said "It's a virus. And a virus is a virus is a virus. So kill it with antivirals." He of course was talking about natural antivirals as they are much broader spectrum than drugs that are designed to target any specific virus. His opinion was that Western doctors were concentrating too much on targeting a specific virus (and a very clever one at that) instead of going for the overall picture – i.e., enhance the immune system and use natural broad-spectrum antivirals. The end.

So when I got Lyme Disease, I thought, "A bacteria is a bacteria is a bacteria. Kill it with antibacterials." And that's what I did. No drugs, no antibiotics, just immune enhancement and natural broad-spectrum antibacterials. After I got rid of it, two things happened. One; this idea I had of going back to school to become a Naturopath actually turned into a reality, and two; this was the final straw and I got the heck out of Nashville. Those ticks are murder.

As you can probably tell, I deal with Lyme Disease a lot. Since almost all of my new clients come to me by referral, I guess it shouldn't shock me to a great degree at how much strangers seem to know about me, but it still takes me by surprise at times. I take phone calls from 9:00-10:00 in the morning. Anyone can call then (time permitting), clients, referrals, people with general questions, and there have been many times when I answered, "This is Shauna, can I help you?", and the first words I hear are, "I heard you once had Lyme Disease."

As a Naturopath, I can't tell you much about what happened with the horde of Lyme's clients I've worked with, but as a private citizen and person who has been-there-done-that-have-the-T-shirt with Lyme's, I *can* tell you what happened with *me*. I had it for four months (four long, rotten, lousy months) and I don't have it anymore. And I haven't had it for 14 years now.

Again, the symptoms of Lyme Disease are multiple and they manifest in numerous ways; it often gets diagnosed as a huge variety of things. Usually what happens initially is that you start to feel generally lousy. Tired, achy joints and muscles, stiff neck, fever, nausea, maybe a sore throat. Sounds a lot like the flu doesn't it? So you take a hot bath, pop a couple of Advil®, and go to bed. You might even start feeling a little better for a while. I've spoken to tons of people who said, "I had the flu for a few days and then it got a little better, but I never felt like I shook it all the way."

The next phase is even more fun. Being tired now turns into this grinding, debilitating fatigue that makes you feel like you're walking hip deep through wet cement. The body aches turn into severely painful joints (especially large joints) and muscle pain, sometimes that includes numbness, tingling or burning in your extremities, or even Bell's palsy. Then comes the ever-wonderful depression, brain fog and lack of bladder control. One client told me that this was so severe for her that she "couldn't keep a thought in her head or an ounce in her bladder for a second." This is common, and a big reason that I get suspicious if someone complains of both fatigue and bladder control issues. Over time, you can add heart, eye, gastrointestinal and respiratory problems, although I wonder if at least some of these may be as much from the antibiotics as the Lyme's.

Strangely enough, with all my book research and time logged on Lyme's websites, there's one symptom I've never seen mentioned, and yet I've rarely seen a Lyme's person who didn't have it. For me it was one of the worst things about the whole ordeal, and when it finally quit happening I knew I was getting better. Every morning I would lie in bed looking at the floor as if it were a pit of snakes, because I knew that as soon as I would get up this same thing would happen. The moment my feet touched the floor, a lightning-like sharp pain would shoot from my feet and go through my body that would feel like it was blowing the top of my head off! I have never felt pain like that in my life, and hope (please, please, please) never to again. Excruciating. Once while talking to a woman about her condition (as yet undiagnosed and currently on hopeful antidepressants) she described this exact pain to me. Since then, I've asked many people about this and it's truly surprising how many reply with a shocked "YES! That's it exactly."

So my last word on Lyme's is this: If you find yourself with a weird undiagnosed condition, or you've been diagnosed with something like chronic fatigue, Fibromyalgia or arthritis and your pills aren't working, you might want to check out some Lyme Disease websites. I'm not *diagnosing* mind you, I'm just saying...

So I can read your mind now. You're wondering what my track record is with these things. Well, you know the answer to that. I can't tell you. But ask yourself this: Would you get on a plane and go halfway around the country (or halfway around the world in the case of some of my clients) if you didn't have a pretty strong recommendation from someone? Think about it. And I'm far from the only natural practitioner working with this kind of stuff.

And oh yes, since I am allowed to talk about my failures, I will tell you that I have had very limited success with the Rockin' Pneumonia and the Boogie-Woogie Flu. Those people just *gotta* dance!

CHAPTER 7

Funny Business

"The truth is that our race survived ignorance; it is our scientific genius that will do us in."

— STEPHEN VIZINCZEY,
BEST SELLING AUTHOR

Working on the scale and at the pace that I do, sometimes it feels like all there is to save me is a sense of humor, and luckily a lot of my clients are very funny people. Some on purpose and some... not so much! Regardless of whether they meant to be or not, a moment to laugh is often a lifesaver. Remember, a wise man once said, "Laughter is the best medicine." I personally think it ranks up there with...water and enzymes!

Much of what they say that I consider funny is about taking the supplements themselves, or in sticking to their diet. It never ceases to amaze me that people can eat horrible food, smoke, drink diet sodas, and take handfuls of prescription drugs, but it's always "the herbs" that have somehow upset their applecarts. Here are some notable examples:

"I know you told me to avoid dairy, but I'm still eating cheese. Is that okay?"

Uh...no. Cheese is dairy. Basic rule of thumb: If an udder was involved anywhere in the process, then it's dairy.

"My diet says I can have apricots. Can I have *chopped* apricots?"

I know it sounds crazy, but I swear to you this has been said to me many, many times (although not always apricots). There is a new eating disorder relatively recently coined called "Orniphobia" that relates to people who have reversed their terrible health problems with diet and are now terrified to mess it up, but I think it's mostly just people not using their heads. To my knowledge, cutting up food doesn't change its nutritional value, although a friend of mine swears that broken cookies don't have any calories.

"After the first three days I stopped taking all the supplements because they were causing my (headaches, diarrhea, insomnia, knee pain, foggy head, funny walk, whatever). How come I don't feel any better?"

Well, let's see. Maybe because you didn't take anything I recommended? For some reason it seems to be a tough thing to get through to some people that it isn't enough to *buy* the supplements, you actually have to *take* them. Strangely enough, this comment is most often made by people who originally came in with the very complaint they say the supplements caused! For example, a woman in her 30's told me that she stopped taking the teas I recommended because they were causing diarrhea, when the reason she came to see me in the first place was that she'd had daily diarrhea for many years! She felt a bit silly when I reminded her of this little detail.

"Do the supplements cause projectile vomiting very often?"

Uh...no. Nope, not ever that I know of. It just slays me to think that someone could think that something like projectile vomiting wouldn't be discussed under the "possible side effects" conversation I have with everyone at the end of their appointments. I have been tempted to say, "Oh yeah, didn't I mention that?" But in the end I found it better to maintain some professionalism.

As I mentioned before (numerous times), one of the biggest challenges facing a Naturopath is to get people to drink enough water. You'd think we were trying to poison them! Although water will be discussed in great length throughout the book, here are a few misconceptions and fears regarding simple H_2O:

"Water makes me gag."

Believe it or not, people actually say this. They can drink coffee, soda, ice tea or scotch, but water makes them gag. I'm sorry, but I find this comment a bit hard to swallow (pun intended). The only time that this is even *close* to being true is with people with severe liver issues. Even though they need water worse than anyone, it is hard at times since the liver damage causes water to taste very coppery, like blood. So although this has been a clue to what we were dealing with in some cases, for the most part the gag-thing is complete hooey.

"I'll have to pee."

Probably. And the problem with that is...? Possibly a toilet paper phobia? The key to not losing all the water you just drank is to take small sips of room temperature water throughout the day. After all, your stomach, bladder and kidneys are holding-tanks of a sort, and can't take too much at once. Give them a little time to absorb! However, yes, peeing will always be part of the process.

"I'll be up all night."

Just like you probably tell your kids, no fluids after a certain hour then. Don't drink all your water just before bed. And when you get sufficiently hydrated, chances are this will stop anyway. One note here: If you do get up in the night, try to not turn on any lights. Light will cause your pineal gland to stop releasing melatonin (a hormone that helps you sleep). Melatonin starts percolating in you when the sun goes down, and stops when it comes up.

"I don't drink any water, but I do drink a lot of coffee and tea. There's water in those, right?"

This one is actually kind of cute. They always say this with their head kind of tilted to one side and very softly with such a hopeful look on their faces – one of those sheepish "I'm sorry" smiles. As a matter of fact, for every coffee, tea or soda you drink, you have to drink extra water to make up for the dehydration caused by those beverages. And to answer the next question, yes, that also applies to decaffeinated products and things to "add to your water" as well. I recently saw a commercial for a low-calorie powdered drink product informing viewers that since you need to drink your water anyway, "why not make your water delicious" or "pump up your water". Not only is this product one of the worst on the market for being loaded with artificial sweeteners (which dehydrate you even further and cause all kinds of other problems), but if you add anything except fruit juice to water, it isn't water anymore. That anyone can even pretend to think this, shows the absolute power of rationalization. I've even had a few people (men) who asked the same about *beer*. Now *that's* the power of rationalization!

Never A Dull Moment

In our office, we don't require the reams of paperwork that many practitioners have. Ours is short and to the point. This is why I find it so strange when some clients don't answer the few, reasonable questions we do pose. For example, we ask how many metal fillings someone has in his or her mouth. This seems like a very straightforward question to me, but we certainly don't get straightforward answers. Instead of saying "3" or "10" or "none", we almost constantly get "some", "a few" or "a bunch". My (least) favorite is, "I don't know", sometimes notated on the paperwork as "?". They actually write down "I don't know." Well, how about go look in the mirror and count! I'll wait here.

We also get a lot of odd answers about stress level. I ask for a number on a scale between 1 and 10. Instead we get, "varies", "a lot", "some", and "matters on what day". Not very helpful for me I can assure you. I guess it just proves once again how different Allopathic and Naturopathic modalities are. We Naturopaths care about things like how much metal lives in your mouth, your stress level, and even whether or not you enjoy your job. I guess they just don't get asked those kinds of questions enough for them to think it matters. It does.

People just being people though, have enriched our office and the jobs we do here. These are just some plain old funny lines that people have said. There have been many, but these in particular stick in my mind:

A late 20's newlywed was worried about her low libido. The mind was willing, but her endometriosis was holding her back. Anything we could do while working on that? So I gave her some Maca to try to increase her testosterone. A few weeks later, her husband came in my office with a tape measurer and without a word to me or anyone, started taking measurements. I asked what he was doing, and he said, "Just trying to figure out where you'll want your statue." I'm thinking the Maca worked.

On the subject of sex, another newlywed couple of about two months came in together. He was 92 and she was 86. He said, "Ya know doc, we may not be kids, but we have sex *almost* every night." I replied, "Really? That's great!" He continued, "Yep. We almost did on Monday, we almost did on Tuesday, we almost did on Wednesday." His wife hates that joke. I love it.

I had a man in his early 60's tell me that he had "congenital diarrhea". When I questioned this he said, "It runs in my jeans."

And speaking of diarrhea, a woman in her 30's had suffered from terrible chronic diarrhea for many years. Before starting her on a parasite cleanse, she asked if she would "see anything". I think she had visions in her head of the awful photos you see on websites from Africa and other countries with twenty pounds of two-foot-long worms coming out. I told her not to worry – in her area if she saw anything, they would probably look like sesame seeds or rice, as they were the "local varieties". A month later she sat in front of me with that I-have-good-news look on her face that I have come to know so well. She said she had good news and bad news: "The good news is, my diarrhea stopped. The bad news is I'll never be able to look a hamburger bun in the face again." I'm thinking she had the sesame-seed-looking variety.

And while on that subject, I finally talked a woman in her 50's into doing a gallbladder flush. People are often shocked at the amount of bright green gallstones they are able to pass without pain and so quickly as a result of doing an effective cleanse. She called me absolutely shocked at how many stones she had passed (around 50 she estimated). Her husband had been leery of her doing the flush (as he is of me, all natural medicine, the media, the government and pretty much everything else), and she wanted to prove to him that it had worked. She told me, "It was the first time in thirty-six years of marriage that I ever yelled, 'Hey come in here and see this!'" Now *that's* a strong marriage!

Many people have asked me this, but I still think it's funny. "Can I use your blood pressure machine? I want to know what it really is and I'm not afraid of you." Just for the record, I also suffer from what many call "White Coat Syndrome" so I understand. This is yet another reason why I have no desire to dress like a doctor, since the briefest glimpse of a white doctor's coat coupled with a cold exam room and that weird smell of a doctor's office (what *is* that anyway?) is enough to blast the blood pressure of most of us skyward just from sheer trepidation.

A remedy I use with nearly everyone is a brand of Essiac that is called Ojibwa Tea (since it is originally an Ojibwa Indian recipe). One of my clients told me that he was taking his supplements and was feeling a lot better, but he also said he'd done some research and found out why the Ojibwa tribe was so unpopular with people. This was news to me, as the Ojibwa are a well-known and highly regarded tribe. He said, "Well, they were always inviting people over for tea." I guess he didn't like its earthy taste as well as I do!

A woman in her mid-50's who had suffered for years from horrible and debilitating knee pain said she knew she was getting better, because she'd been able to go to "a wonderful place I haven't been able to get to for years." When I asked where this exotic locale was, she said, "The upstairs of my house." Good thing she's not allergic to dust!

A Candida detox, while a very necessary thing, can be decidedly un-fun. The detox symptoms range from person to person and from negligible to pretty severe. For most, the symptoms cycle in and out as yeast builds up then is dumped, then builds again, and people's energy has a tendency to be a bit of a rollercoaster ride at times until it clears out. While many have tried to describe this feeling to me, my favorite was one client who said her energy went from quite low to extremely high. She called her high days "Julie Andrews days, where I just want to dance across mountaintops and sing!" I have used the term "Julie Andrews days" to many people since. They seem to all instantly know what I'm talking about.

And here's my favorite. Clients often ask me to research products for them, as there are so many out there making claims to address everything from joint pain, to gray hair, to making you irresistible to the opposite sex. The one she asked me to investigate was definitely in this mode, going on and on for pages about its benefits and loaded with glowing testimonials. Apparently a few drops of this fabulous elixir would cure everything that could be wrong or ever would go wrong with you. When I called her back, I told her of my doubts that anything could possibly do all that. In her priceless Texas drawl she said, "Yeah, it does look like a few drops of this stuff would turn a cow pie into a cinnamon roll." From that moment on, the code word in my office for anything too good to be true was and remains "cinnamon roll".

Just so no one thinks I'm poking fun at them, I'll rat myself out on my worst ever faux pas. As I mentioned already, my sense of humor has a tendency to be on the dark and dry side at times anyway, and it gets darker the more tired I become. At the end of a very long day that fell at the end of a very long week, a man and his wife came in to see me. He was a Vietnam War vet with high blood pressure, high cholesterol, obesity and massive back and body pains. As I looked through his list of the thirteen, yes *thirteen* prescription medications he was taking (three of them mind numbing and highly addictive narcotic painkillers), I saw one I didn't understand; a very strong antipsychotic drug. In response to my question of why he was taking it, he told me that he also had a diagnosis of Post-Traumatic Stress Disorder, and that he heard voices in his head. Without thinking (obviously) I responded with, "I hope they tell you when to take your pills." Silence. Dead silence.

As I kept my eyes downcast and locked on his chart madly trying to think of a good enough apology (to this *date* I still haven't thought of one), he and his wife looked at each other in shock. Instead of hurling himself across my desk to throttle me as he had every right to do, they started to laugh. And laugh. And *laugh*. When he could breathe again, he told me that he had been dragged into my office against his will by his wife (a common lament from husbands), but now felt glad to be here. He thought that "Anyone with the brass to say something like that must know what they're doing", and suddenly felt relaxed. It was totally my good luck that it worked out well, but from then on I've been much more careful about what I say. The next guy might not have such a good sense of humor! Incidentally, the voices in his head turned out to be from the painkillers, not Vietnam.

My irreverent sense of humor did once drive a husband out of my office. A couple in their 60's came in one day. When I asked why they were here, he snapped, "She needs her sex drive fixed." On questioning, he seemed to feel that her libido was rather low (I always ask now whether it's too high or too low because I've been caught on that one a time or two). Before trying to "fix" her to his satisfaction, I asked a few questions. While he had retired not long ago, she was still working full time. "Okay. So when she gets home from work, you have dinner waiting for her?" I asked. His gruff answer was "I don't cook." The rest of the questions I asked elicited the same basic answer. Apparently, though retired with much more time on his hands than her, he did not shop, cook, clean house, do laundry or wash dishes.

By this time he was getting very agitated. She on the other hand was pinching herself and covering her mouth so she wouldn't laugh. I summed up, "So she stops on the way home after eight to ten hours at work to shop, cook dinner, clean up after it then does some housework or laundry after dinner. You on the other hand, don't shop, cook, clean or help her in any way, yet you expect her to want to have sex with you? To my knowledge there's no pill for that." The dam blew, and she burst out laughing. He just burst out, period. He never came in again. His wife, however, has been a loyal client since then. She and I still laugh about that sometimes. Sex?? I'm surprised she even *speaks* to him.

Sometimes too, the powers that be do work in mysterious ways. Like the man who inadvertently gave me the title for this book. This poor guy had suffered from a terrible, itching rash that for about five months had been spreading progressively all over his body like some evil tidal wave. One morning, he woke up with hives on his back and despite multiple appointments with multiple "specialists" this demonic rash was getting continually worse. He was taking five prescription medications for allergies, anxiety and hives, as well as three different steroid injections. He was miserable and was told that he'd be like that "for the rest of his life." He was only 63 and a pretty robust and active dude, so that prognosis held little appeal for him. After asking my usual questions, I found out he'd worked in chemical plants and oil fields all his life. Can you say…toxic blood?

A few months later he was off all prescriptions and the hives were completely gone. The timing was unfortunate for his doctor's office – this was when they called to tell him to come in for his steroid injections. He politely told them that he didn't need any injections, that his hives were all gone and thanks for checking. The nurse got, in his words "very huffy" and told him "That was impossible." He told her that he was currently *living* in his skin and knew for a fact that it didn't have any hives on it. She asked how that could be possible, and he told her that he had gone out to Colorado to see a Naturopath he'd been referred to, and his rash and hives had gone away under her care. The nurse's incredulous (but oh so inspiring for me) answer: "That's impossible! Naturopaths are quacks!"

I guess I don't have to tell you what he said.

CHAPTER 8

Weird Cases, or "Miracles Do Happen"

"There are no such things as incurable, there are only things for which man has not found a cure."

— BERNARD MANNES BARUCH,
U.S. FINANCIER AND PRESIDENTIAL ADVISOR

I confess: "Weird" is my specialty. Weird could be my middle name, although I'm glad it isn't because I rather like the whole "SKY" thing my parents did, and that would make it "SWY" instead. Face it, you just don't get on a plane to go see some Naturopath you've been referred to unless what you've got is pretty weird. Ergo, my specialty.

In truth, most Naturopaths don't get to have a specialty. People often ask me (like I'm a regular doctor or something), "So what's your specialty?" When you view and work with the body as a whole, it becomes hard to specialize in any given part of it. Even if I decided to become, say, an allergy specialist, or an arthritis specialist, I'd still have to know how to do all the stuff I do now, so what's the point? Because as I've said before, we don't treat symptoms, we work with causes and with fortifying and balancing your immune system. And while it's true that the cause of one person's allergies and another person's arthritis may be Candida in both cases, it's also true that the cause of one person's arthritis may be totally different from the cause for another person who is also suffering from arthritis.

Whew. You may want to read that last sentence over slowly a few times. I had to. For example, I've always found the "ear, nose and throat" specialty interesting, since we find that most of the symptoms that manifest in your ear, nose or throat originate in your bowel. However, we already discussed the whole bowel thing in another chapter, so I'll leave that alone for now, for which I'm sure you're grateful. A little bowel talk goes a long way.

Since we encounter the oxymoron of "everyday miracles" so much around here, it was a challenge for me to decide which cases to present in this chapter. As an FYI, my definition of "everyday miracles" are the cases that, although they were fairly straightforward in my mind, brought a result that was miraculous *to the client*. This happens pretty often when you detox someone of nasties like parasites, Candida or artificial sweeteners, and all their symptoms that have bothered them for years often just – whoosh! – vanish in a fairly short period of time. It *seems* like a miracle to the person who had the migraines, skin condition, joint or abdominal pain, depression or whatever, but it is also the exact result I expected to happen when the immune system clocks in and starts doing its job. What I am presenting here are some of the cases that stand out the most to me and have stayed clear in my mind over the years.

A Very Unusual Christmas Present

Although this case is a fairly run-of-the-mill example of what happens with a Candida detox, it stands out strongly to me because of the lesson she taught me.

Although only in her very early 50's, this woman had received a diagnosis of rheumatoid arthritis more than 20 years prior. She'd seen multiple doctors (including a few natural ones) and had been on various pain medications, none of which had helped, including one that is also a *chemotherapy* drug that is sometimes used on arthritis. So now she was on an anti-depressant in the hopes, I had supposed, that her symptoms were all mental, or at least that she'd keep more quiet about them. However, there was nothing mental about her spastic colon caused by the variety of medications she'd been taking. She was unable to even get on a plane because of it, and consequently had not even been able to meet her new grandchild.

My first clue that she was not suffering from arthritis was that the arthritis pain medications hadn't worked. One positive thing you can say about pharmaceuticals is that when it comes to effectively masking symptoms, they work! So if you're taking an arthritis pill and it doesn't work, it's a pretty safe bet that you don't have arthritis. So, in describing her symptoms, she gave a textbook description (my textbook anyway) of systemic Candida albicans: Joint pain, spastic colon, reflux, ringing in her ears, rashes, depression – the whole ball of wax – or ball of yeast as the case may be. So we started a routine Candida detox.

A month later, after sticking meticulously to her dietary and supplement protocol, she reported dramatic results. Her spastic colon symptoms had all but disappeared, and for the first time in more than 20 years, she had been pain free for a whole week from her "arthritis" symptoms. Needless to say, she was pretty happy! After a few more months of work, I discharged her and didn't expect to see her for another year.

She came in a few months later at Christmas time, telling me she had a present for me, and wanted to go into my office to give it to me. Instead of the more traditional fruitcake I was expecting, she gave me a large Ziploc® bag filled with what appeared to be pills of various kinds. At my blank look, she said, "I wanted to show these to you, because I don't need them anymore." "Oh, I get it" I said, "These are all your old pain pills your doctor took you off and you no longer need." Odd gift, but I got the point. Or so I thought.

As it happened, they weren't just her old pain pills. They were pills that she had been collecting for years. She had gotten them mostly as samples from doctors, although some were from other people's medicine cabinets. I was still in the dark, so she elaborated. Tired of her never-ending pain and ever-escalating symptoms, she had been collecting them in order to more effectively kill herself. She had a whole collection of different types so that no one in the emergency room could figure out what she'd taken and antidote it (a tidbit she learned from an episode of a television show). I had been her "last resort" before using them. That phrase again. I had no way of knowing how often I'd hear it over the coming years.

Stunned does not begin to describe how I felt. As I sat there, holding this big bag of pills, I didn't know what to feel. New to the business as I was, I have to admit that my first thought was thank goodness the detox had worked. What if I had worked with her, then learned that she had committed suicide! She laughed at my stunned face, and said "Relax. I don't want them anymore. That's why I'm giving them to you." Then she stood up, wished me a Merry Christmas and was gone.

Still a bit shell-shocked, I sat in my office looking at this bomb in a Ziploc®. My Mom (who worked with me at the time) came in, and when she saw the bag, asked what it was. "Poison" was the only response I could come up with.

It was the oddest Christmas present I have ever received, and the *only* one I've ever flushed down a toilet, yet it taught me a very important lesson that I never have forgotten, and never will. Although her case seemed straightforward, even "easy" for me, it was paramount to her. I learned at that moment to always look at the situation from the client's perspective, not my own. And that is still, to this day, the way I practice. And I thank her from my heart for teaching me that very important lesson so early on. Truly, there are no accidents.

The "No-name" Syndromes

My first client who actually had to fly in to see me was a 56-year-old carpenter who was on disability. His sister, who was one of my clients, had "made him come". He had been in a severe car wreck four years earlier, which had required several rounds of surgery, antibiotics and x-rays. Already I knew what was coming, although in his case it was necessary. Antibiotics and x-rays are a disastrous combination. The antibiotics kill the friendly bowel flora allowing the Candida to grow out of control then the radiation from the x-rays causes it to bloom like some hideous garden. And unfortunately, once Candida becomes systemic in your body it loses its marker in a blood test, making it very difficult to detect on a standard test. He presented the usual suspects in Candida cases: Joint and muscle pain, fatigue, weakness, chronic bronchitis, depression and digestive issues.

During our conversation, his sister left the room for a moment. The second she walked out, he quickly leaned forward and almost whispered, "I got something I need to tell you." Obviously something he didn't want his sister to hear. "I think I'm going crazy. I feel like I've got something crawling around inside of me, like an alien or something." He was rather relieved when I told him that actually, he was very accurate. He did indeed have something alien alive inside him.

What a lot of people don't realize about Candida (and other microbes, parasites, etc.) is that they are *alive*. And anything alive has its own agenda, and that is to *stay* alive and to grow. When you are waging a battle against Candida or parasites, understand that they are fighting back! Sugar feeds all kinds of viruses, yeasts, molds and parasites, and they love it, so they'll literally make you crave sugar so they can grow and thrive. When you try to put something in your body to kill them, they react and react hard, and you need to be ready for it. When I warned him that his Candida would stage a revolt when we went to kill it, he admitted (as many people have) that his sugar cravings were already so strong that he was waking up in the night craving sugar. Understanding why you crave sugar so strongly goes a long way toward being able to resist it.

Although he was very dubious that a mere fungus could do such damage, he was in such pain that he was willing to try anything. A carpenter by trade, he was unable to even bend his fingers. We made sure he had enough supplements to last him for a while, and he went back home.

When I spoke to him a month later, he was a different person. His pain was still with him a bit, but it had lifted to the point that he was going off disability and soon, back to work. He described his progress as "drastic" and that he could see "daily improvement". As in the case described above, it was the progress that I had rather expected, although admittedly his was more rapid then usual. He saw it as a miracle. He continued his detox and his health continued to improve.

The funny part of this story for me was the reaction of his doctors after he went back to work. The State where he lives is one of those "licensed states" I previously mentioned where the practice of Traditional Naturopathy is a felony. I had to be very careful when his doctors started contacting me. One of them actually called me in person rather than sending yet another letter. He first stated that he couldn't believe the improvement he'd seen and that he had previously doubted if this gentleman would ever be off disability. Now for the tricky part. He asked me, "So what was your diagnosis?" I explained to him that I am a Naturopath and therefore do not diagnose. "Okay" he said, "Then what did you treat him for?" That, I could answer: "Systemic Candida."

Silence. "What?" he asked. "Systemic Candida Albicans", I said again. More silence. He cleared his throat, "No let me clarify. What exactly were you working with him for?" Again, my answer, "Systemic Candida."

It was easy to see where this was going, and that's exactly where it went. He kept asking me in different ways what we'd worked on, and I kept giving him the same answer. It was as if I was speaking Venutian and he was speaking Martian; we were just not on the same page. I kept telling him what I did, and he kept not accepting it as an issue since it wasn't a "diagnosis". We started to sound like a medical version of Abbot and Costello's "Who's on First?" In the end, I referred him to a website that discussed the issues created by excess Candida. It seems that in order for something to be an *illness*, it has to have a *name*. Hopefully someone in the medical industry will put his or her personal name to this issue and coin a term for systemic Candida, so that doctors will recognize and diagnose it. All I know is that I'd hate to have it named after me!

Miracle or...?

I'll be honest with you; like many other cases, I have no idea how this one worked. I didn't then and I don't really now. I'm just glad it worked for this sweet little boy.

Early on in my practice, a very scared Mom brought in her eight-year-old son. His epilepsy had started at about six months of age, and despite medication upon medication his seizures had become progressively worse. His Mother was extremely worried about his liver since he was taking massive adult doses of both Tegretol® and Adderall® (look those two up in the PDR if you want a good scare). Sadly, despite the heavy doses of these very strong anti-seizure meds, he was still having multiple cluster seizures daily.

By now I was using a bio-resonant testing device within my assessment process, and although the output still does not constitute a *diagnosis*, it pointed in this case to the possibility of a massive amount of parasites in his system – more than I had ever seen, or quite honestly, imagined. I was totally honest with his Mother. I told her that my experience specifically with epilepsy was limited, but I felt strongly that we needed to do some restorative work on his liver, and above all, get rid of those parasites. I also promised that I would do research on seizures and see if there was anything we could do naturally to help. His mother left feeling that at least we were doing something positive for him. The years of seizures and drugs had taken their toll on the poor kid and his Mom.

Fortunately, kids bounce fast. A mere two weeks after we started his parasite detox, his Mother called to tell me that her son's seizures had stopped. The first few days were "terrible" (again, the bugs putting up a fight), but then he abruptly started settling down. He had only had one small seizure since the fourth day of detox. The last time he had gone for an entire day without seizures was *three years prior*, representing over a third of his young life. About a month and a half later, his medical doctor took him off all his prescription drugs and he remained seizure free.

Why? I have very little idea. Even though people like Hulda Clark recognized how often parasites are the culprit in a myriad of illnesses, this still seemed extreme. Two weeks? He went from daily multiple seizures to none in two weeks? It still blows my mind. Although he hated his supplements at first, he quickly grew to love them, often reminding his busy Mother to give him his "black juice" (the black walnut, wormwood and clove tincture that kills parasites) and his "fish herbs" (EPA's). This one, even to me, was a miracle indeed.

A Bird in a Cage

When I'm having one of those "Ah what's the use" days, I can think of this girl and remember why I keep at it. This lovely young lady came in not long after I opened my practice, and her success is still continuing to unfold. It just keeps getting better.

One of the saddest things any health care professional deals with is the "CP Kids". Cerebral Palsy is a brutal disease caused by damage or trauma to the brain that affects muscle coordination, movement and balance. Over 3,000 infants are born with cerebral palsy in this country every year, while another 500 a year will develop the condition in early childhood. It is considered incurable. While it is not fatal and the condition doesn't progress, it is devastating for the child and wreaks havoc on the lives of his or her family. It is mentally, emotionally and physically draining, and the medical expenses alone can be staggering. This poor kid was no exception.

At the time she came in with her exhausted Mom and Dad, she was 15 years old and had spent all of her years in a wheelchair unable to move or speak. In addition to the wheelchair, she was held up by an additional strap across her chest, as she was unable to hold her head or upper body upright. She had almost no movement in her arms or legs. At first I was a bit puzzled as to why her parents had brought her in to our office, so they explained that all they were looking for was some relief for the uncomfortable side effects like constipation, weight gain, pressure sores and the like; all resulting from being wheelchair bound.

After hooking her up to my test equipment, I got several surprises one after the other. For one thing, she was showing every sign of extreme brain activity, and in fact "frustration" showed up a lot. What was also apparent was the possibility of massive skull damage. I was very puzzled. I also felt hog-tied. Prohibited from diagnosing, I had to find a way of clearly communicating these suspicions without contradicting anyone. Finally, I just said, "Is there any possibility that the back of her skull got damaged somehow?" Her Mom and Dad exchanged a meaningful and miserable glance. Uh oh. I waited.

Very painfully, with his wife holding his hand for support, her Dad started to tell the story. She was a premature baby, and the delivery (with him in the room) was a frightening and brutal experience. As he described the scene, the doctors, in his words "tore" the baby out of his wife, "slammed" her on a table, "jerked" back her head (so much that he heard cracking and popping) and "shoved" an intubation tube down her throat. He yelled at them to stop, "Hey, that's a baby!" He was told that it was "going to be a dead baby" if they didn't get her intubated (which was quite possible, but why the force?), and took him, protesting, out of the delivery room. As he was telling this awful story, he was getting more and more (understandably) upset. He finished with tears rolling down his face and saying he "still had nightmares" about it sometimes.

His wife was watching him, but I was watching his daughter. The whole time he was talking, she was quite agitated. As her Father got more and more upset, her "random" movements started to look not so random to me. She kept trying very purposefully to manipulate her arm so that she could get her hand onto her Father's arm. She just kept at it, until finally her hand flopped onto his wrist. She was trying to comfort him! This was not the usual M.O. for a CP child. She was showing unmistakable sympathy for him.

Under the guise of getting her Dad some water, I took her parents out of the room. I told them that there were things that could be done for the constipation, weight and so on, but I asked if they had ever heard of cranial sacral therapy; a very delicate type of bodywork (I think of it more as an art form) that very gently manipulates the bones of the skull. Fortunately for us (in our little area) we had a world-class cranial sacral therapist in a nearby town – oddly enough, the very same town this family lived in.

They were interested. I refrained from saying what I thought it might do, I just suggested they try it. I also asked them to go on the web and look up some information on hyperbaric oxygen therapy (HBOT). They agreed to do both, very excited about the fact that someone was actually suggesting at least *something* they could try.

As they went out to the front desk, I went in alone and spoke to their teenager. I took both her hands, and leaned down so that I could look her in the eye. I said, "Let me tell you what *I* think. I think you understand every word we've said; in fact, I think you always do. I think that if your brain could just figure out the right pathways, that you could tell us what's on your mind. I think that there is a sweet and smart kid in there, and I'm going to do everything I can think of to help get you out of there. Okay?" The gratitude in her eyes with the tears leaking from them told me that I was on the right track. I just had to find a way to get that child out of her cage. I couldn't say that to anyone else, but in that moment I promised myself to live up to those words.

After speaking to the therapist at length, her parents decided to try the cranial sacral therapy for their daughter. A couple months later, she started to talk. She didn't have a lot of facility at first, but the vocabulary was there. My hunch had been right. She had understood everything anyone had said to her all along – her brain just wasn't getting the right signals to let her speak. At this point, we found a hyperbaric chamber for them to try. I am a big believer in HBOT for oxygen deficiencies, and her poor brain had been oxygen-starved for a long time.

After a while, she got such good result from the treatments, and she was gaining so much more ability of movement that her parents decided to buy a hyperbaric chamber to keep in their home. Wanting to speed her progress as much as possible, she got in the chamber for an hour every day. From there on, her improvement was hard to believe.

As this could turn into a very long story, I'll hit the high points. At 16, she was mainstreamed into high school. She was bright, happy and made a lot of new friends. When she graduated with her class, she won a state-wide high school award in psychology. I asked her how she got so smart, and she told me (very matter-of-a-factly) that "When you don't speak for 15 years, you have a lot of time to think." Good point. Over the years she has told me many wise things; she's quite a gal.

One day I had to ask her the inevitable question. Was she ever bitter about what had happened to her? She thought about it a long time before answering, then said "No, not really. It wasn't any fun, but if it hadn't happened I never would have known what lengths my whole family would go to for me. My parents, my grandparents, they gave up their whole lives to try to make mine better. They'd do anything in the world for me. How many people get to know that? I can do anything with that kind of support behind me."

And she is. As of this writing, she is 21 and taking psychology classes at the local college campus here. She isn't walking yet, but she does take yoga classes and says walking is next. The way she puts it is "I have to walk. I want to buy a car." I'm certainly not going to question it! She's certainly done everything else she has said she would do. She has a great family, great physical therapists, and most important, a great attitude. Sometimes, it's all about faith.

As for school, she's doing great. I think that psychology is a good path for her as she understands things that most of us never will, mostly because we never had to. But one thing is for absolute certain: This golden bird is well and truly out of her cage.

Sweet Poison

This one I include not so much for the case itself, but because I've seen so many like this. Most people have heard that artificial sweeteners are a problem, but in my mind few are taking the dangers of them seriously enough. People forget that the original artificial sweeteners were released onto the market as ant poisons (they work very well for that by the way), and they are serious and potentially deadly neurotoxins. It was only after it was discovered that they were so sweet and calorie-free that they were declassified as "poison" and reclassified as a "dietary ingredient". Talk about an inconvenient truth! I wonder who had that original bright idea. Yuck. And wouldn't you love to have the money the companies had to pay out to reclassify poisons into food additives without changing the formulas? Bet that was a chunk of change.

Most folks remember to avoid diet sodas well enough, but they don't avoid packaged drink mixes, nearly all gums and breath mints (unless you get them at the health food store, they're probably loaded with artificial sweeteners), nearly all regular market toothpastes and mouthwashes; unfortunately, this list goes on and on. It's terrible, and they're in everything. It helps to be a good label reader, but even if you are, there are still ways to hide them. For example, toothpaste only has to list "active ingredients" and are allowed to leave out all the others; the "others" often being things such as artificial sweeteners and aluminum. No big.

One crazy experience I had with this stuff took place in the Las Vegas airport. I travel a lot and I like to chew gum when I fly to keep my ears equalized, so I went into a gift shop to buy some gum. The gum and mints counter was about the size of a '69 Buick with a jillion choices, so I figured surely I could find something without aspartame, Splenda® or Nutrasweet® in it, right? Wrong. I was first bewildered at the additives in gum (why would you need sugar *and* aspartame?), then moved on to being appalled, and finally it turned into a quest. After the sales person asked me for the hundredth time, with more and more exasperation apparent each time if she could help me, I stopped answering her and kept right on obsessively reading labels. I finally found one thing without listed artificial sweeteners: Tic Tac®. That's it. It brought home to me (once again) how prevalent and insidious the use of this stuff is, and how hard it is to avoid.

Admittedly some people are more sensitive to these chemicals than others, but we will all become truly intoxicated from them over time. So if you think you're probably okay on this issue, but you're not positive, do something for me that I like to do at seminars. Go and get your tube of toothpaste and read what's on the label. Most likely it will list some type of fluoride (a carcinogen by the way) as the "active ingredient", but see what else it lists. The one I have sitting on my keyboard at the moment says exactly this (including the bold typeface):

"**WARNING: Keep out of the reach of children under 6 years of age**. If you accidentally swallow more than used for brushing, seek professional assistance or contact a Poison Control Center immediately."

Really! Go on and check it out yourself. I'll wait here again.

You're back? Good. Yowzah! Do you really want to put something in your mouth and that therefore gets under your tongue (the most absorbable spot in your body) twice a day that carries that kind of warning? I don't! My toothpaste comes from the health food store and there is nothing even smacking of a warning on the label. In fact, since mine says that it is "pure, natural and organic" it has to list *all* ingredients, including water, not just the "active" ones. This is a good thing to remember when buying *any* food product: If it isn't making a claim of "pure" or "natural" or "organic", it doesn't always have to disclose all that's in it.

It was one freaked-out teenager who came in with her Mom one day. The only thing worse than the sudden onset of her issues, was the diagnosis she had been handed one month before coming in. According to her she woke up one morning and the whole left side of her body was numb. It got a little better in the next week, but she was into quite a round of tests to try to figure out what was going on. With the discovery of lesions on her brain, she was unceremoniously handed a dreaded diagnosis: Multiple Sclerosis. In addition to the neurological symptoms of tingling, numbness, twitching and headaches, she had another that encouraged me to ask questions about her use of artificial sweeteners. She told me that she was chronically thirsty, even to the point of feeling "desperate for water" at times. This is classic with artificial sweetener toxicity.

We started her on a program that included a homeopathic artificial sweetener detox. An MRI she had less than a month later revealed that her lesions were almost completely healed. According to her Mom, the radiologist hazarded a new diagnosis of sorts: "Maybe not MS." Not conclusive, but not bad.

Am I trying to say that all MS is caused by artificial sweeteners? Of course not. Neither are the groups of symptoms that get diagnosed as Parkinson's, migraines, Fibromyalgia, arthritis, diabetes, depression, Alzheimer's, ADD or epilepsy, but I have seen people with those various "diagnoses" who lost the symptoms when detoxed from and remained off artificial sweeteners.

Maybe the strangest case of such toxicity I ever saw was a woman who had already seen multiple specialists and neurologists with no result by the time she came in to see me. She was painful to even look at as her face was continually twitching and jerking, but it was nothing compared to the pain she was dealing with. When I asked if it hurt, she described the pain as feeling like "a hot match head" on her skin each time it twitched, and she was having continual vicious headaches. When I expressed sympathy as to how that must be to live with, she said, "Try sleeping with the skin crawling off your face and scalp all the time." Fortunately for her, the symptoms were essentially gone in less than a month, and completely gone shortly after that. Even now (several years later) they have not reoccurred.

The thing to keep in mind is that these ubiquitous artificial substances are not harmless non-calorie sweeteners. They are potentially deadly neurotoxins that should be avoided at all costs if you care about your health. And the one that claims it's "made from sugar", isn't. It's made from chlorine. There are 3 chlorine molecules to each 1 of sugar. And the reason it doesn't have calories is because *your body can't digest it*! Again, look it up yourself.

Common Sense

There's a precious thing that is very often overlooked and yet is the number-one tool of the Naturopath. Simple, down-to-earth, everyday, common sense. As I've already said in this book, it is the true basis of natural medicine. If it doesn't make sense, it probably isn't right. Here is a prime example.

This nice 47-year-old (formerly very active) guy came all the way from South Dakota to see me on the advice of his sister, who is one of my clients. He had some of the "usual symptoms" I see often – digestive issues, acid reflux, aches and pains, colitis, along with one very *un*usual symptom. For reasons no one had quite figured out, his lungs had become attached by adhesions to his chest wall! When I asked for more information on this, he opened the top of his shirt and showed me. When he attempted to take a deep breath, you could see the adhesions actually sticking and pulling his skin where they were healed to his chest wall. As you can imagine, this was a very painful and limiting condition. Especially when he was trying to sleep. Or walk. Or breathe. Then I got the hideous news that he'd been dealing with this for *more than 7 years*, with the current treatment suggestion from his doctors being for him to "get some psychotherapy to help him learn to live with the pain." Not an extremely exciting prospect for a young guy with six kids.

The other tough thing for this guy was that it was very obvious that he'd been dragged in here by his sister and wife. He'd been to so many other doctors (both Allopathic and Naturopathic) that he was, justifiably, very skeptical. Fortunately, I am rather used to dealing with skeptical clients, so this didn't bother me too much.

So instead of over-thinking the whole thing, I just thought; what breaks adhesions loose? Enzymes of course! One of the main functions of certain enzymes is that they eat scar tissue, fibrin and adhesions. I explained to him the process of how and why enzymes dissolve scar tissue, and he listened attentively. I then recommended some things to work on his colitis and re-flux, and suggested he take a very large dose of my enzyme complex on an empty stomach to go after the adhesions themselves.

It seemed at first that he was having trouble with the fact that all I was asking him to do was take some capsules that worked on dissolving scar tissue. After all the doctors, the surgeries, the specialists and the tens of thousands of dollars he'd spent over the years, I was saying, "Here, take these capsules. They eat scar tissue." He kept saying, "And that's it, huh?" And I'd say, "Yep. That's it". We did that a bunch of times. He just couldn't believe he'd come all this way, and all I was saying to him was something that simple. You have scar tissue. Take something that works on scar tissue.

He was believing it a whole lot better a few months later when he was able to breathe, sleep and even work out on an elliptical exercise machine without pain. It took a while to get his lungs back into shape, but the feeling of "a thousand needles sticking into me when I try to breathe" was gone pretty quickly, and he, of course, healed a lot faster now that he was able to sleep.

His new question to me was one I couldn't answer: "All the specialists, all the years, all the money. Why didn't anyone else think of this before?" Truthfully, I don't know, dude. It just seemed like common sense to me.

The Big C... or... not

Since this case is actually still in the process of unfolding completely, I hesitated as to whether or not to include it in this book. At the last minute I did decide to add it in because I feel that the story it tells is so vitally and vastly important. So here goes...

Most people feel that the worst news they can possibly receive is that they have "The Big C", and yet cancer diagnoses aren't even unusual anymore and this nice 60 year old lady had already been handed that news... twice. First in 2004 with CLL (Chronic Lymphocytic Leukemia) and then again in 2005 with Non-Hodgkin's Lymphoma, which they treated with both surgery and chemotherapy.

By September of 2010, her white blood cell count (WBC) was starting to rise again and she was looking for some answers. At this point she was feeling increasingly exasperated with the news that her leukemia was on the move with no one ever able to come up with any ideas as to why it was happening. If she didn't know what was causing it, then how could she prevent it? Her daughter-in-law is one of my clients, and finally with her urging (constant pestering) she had decided to make the trip all the way from North Carolina to see if I could come up with anything new.

When I asked about the status of her CLL, she said "They're watching it" and would do more chemo when the WBC numbers warranted it. She was not under any form of treatment and no one had recommended any changes (dietary or otherwise) or anything else for that matter. To be clear, I asked "So they're just going to track you getting sicker and do nothing in the meantime to prevent it?" She heaved a big sigh and said "That's about the size of it." No wonder she wound up in *my* office...

During my initial consultation with her, she told me that she was feeling just fine in general, aside from some chronic sinus issues and a desire to lose some weight. As is usually the case, her CLL was diagnosed using a routine blood test and she never did have any symptoms. Since I've mentioned that, does this seem odd to anyone but me that someone could have cancer and yet still feel good? CLL is the most diagnosed form of leukemia, and yet in most cases it produces no symptoms. This has always seemed strange to me, and since this particular case I've questioned it to an even greater degree.

According to Wikipedia.org (and other sources, but I'm quoting here), "Most people are diagnosed without symptoms as the result of a routine blood test that returns a high white blood cell count...". As it "progresses" it can result in swollen lymph nodes, spleen and liver and eventually anemia and infections. Again quoting Wikipedia, "Early CLL is not treated, and late CLL is treated with Chemotherapy and monoclonal antibodies." Not treated? In other words, no investigation into why a person's white blood cell counts would soar, but just jump right to the extreme solution of *shutting their immune system down* so that the number from the test goes down when it gets "too high". So here's another question: If a person has chemo and their WBC number looks better, will they still be without symptoms, or will they now be suffering from the side effects of the chemo?

So back to my case story. While I was getting this lady prepared for her BioBaseLine® Assessment to supply me with some additional clues, I was thinking about her sinus woes. In my experience (being more than a decade at that time) I have found that truly chronic sinus problems very often result from undetected and/or unresolved dental issues, and sure enough, there were definite dental markers showing up in the assessment. She returned to North Carolina armed with immune system boosters, some detox homeopathics, a truck load of dietary recommendations and a suggestion to see her dentist.

Over the next couple of months I had to conduct follow up appointments by phone since she lived so far away. She was feeling great, losing weight and exercising. Her next blood test was in December. Her WBC count had gone up to 62.25 from being somewhere in the 50's in her last test ("normal" is 4.00 to 11.00) and her platelet count was up to 138. Her doctor was still "watching it". He also told her that if she didn't get a flu vaccine she would "probably die". She decided to take her chances and just say no to the flu shot. The things that some doctors say to people never cease to amaze me.

In January her WBC numbers went up again to 65.1. It seemed as if the immune system enhancers she was taking might be making the count go higher, not lower, which made me even more suspicious of a dental infection being the source of the high WBC results. The problem was that she'd been to the dentist and he had told her there was no problem. Hmm...

In February she again rose to 75.98. She still was feeling great, exercising daily, losing weight and everyone was telling her how great she looked. At this point I urged her to consider thermography testing. Unlike an x-ray (which she'd already had) a thermography produces full color test results that locate and quantify heat and inflammation. I have seen this non-invasive radiation-free test be extremely helpful in revealing covert infections. I gave her the names of three clinics that were closest to her, and she said she'd look into it.

Her March tests were no better – WBC now up to 77.36. Despite this, all she could talk about is how great she felt! She'd been traveling, walking, biking, swimming, anything she wanted. I asked if she was having any trouble with fever or her blood not clotting, and she laughed. In her last blood test they had actually had to repeat it because her blood clotted in the vial! Not a problem usually associated with leukemia…

April and May held more strange results. Her white blood cell count continued to rise, reaching 108.38 in May, and yet her platelet numbers were also rising, not falling as expected. Her oncologist declared himself "non-plussed", which is probably as close to "totally confused" as he was willing to go. As for me, I was still rooting for the idea that it was a dental issue making her WBC numbers rise as her body fought ever harder to rid itself of the infection. On this idea, I recommended some natural antibacterials and antioxidants that she could hold in her mouth before swallowing to see if that would put a dent the WBC numbers. I asked her again about the thermography and she said "Maybe in June".

In June we finally got some results we were looking for. Her count dropped (for the first time) to 103.7. Not a huge drop, but a drop! Maybe we were onto something now. After dropping again to 102.9, her oncologist declared her "stable". At this point I was still campaigning for thermography, but her husband was pushing for a trip to St. John. He won.

The next call in August was not good. Her WBC, which was supposed to be "stable" had soared back up to 127.1. My first question was if in her travels she had stayed consistent with the supplement I suggested for her mouth. As I suspected, her answer was no. Despite the disappointing spike in her WBC, at least the idea of a covert dental infection now seemed more possible to her.

Ten days later she got her thermography. In this form of test results, the color red indicates pretty extreme inflammation, and I'll never forget opening the envelope with a copy of her thermography report. There was bright flaming red extending from her jaw, into her sinus, and to the lymph nodes in both her throat and collar bone area! Wow! Can you say extreme infection? The test interpretation stated "There is hyperthermia around the mouth L>R which may indicate dental/oral pathology". Ya think??

By the end of September her WBC count was up to 152.1 and the plan was on to get her some dental work. On October 12, based on the information provided by the thermography, her oral surgeon found what he described as a "massive infection" under a tooth that apparently didn't seem to have anything wrong with it. When they decided to extract a wisdom tooth on the lower left where all the inflammation was located on the thermograph, this innocent looking tooth let loose a flow of infection that took several days to finish cleaning out. Bingo!

Her WBC test just a few days later showed a drop down to 148.5 just as we expected. Surely it would just continue to drop now that she had evacuated a river of infection from her jaw.

It didn't.

At the end of December her WBC had gone up to 171.8. As you can imagine, she felt "sucker punched" by these new numbers, and as for me, it was now my turn to be "non-plussed" (totally confused). Again, she reported feeling "great". How could that be?

In January her count went up to 202 and she gave me the news I had been expecting (dreading). Even though physically she felt great, she had made the decision to go ahead and undergo more chemo to try to get the numbers down. This is one of the worst parts of this work for me. Although every cell in my body was screaming, "No! No! Please don't flood your body with more poison!", I can't legally say anything of the sort. What I did do was tell her *why* the WBC numbers go down with chemo – because it kills your immune system and your body stops fighting so hard. I also told her my idea as to why the numbers were going up and not down. I suspected that when all that infection was freed from its hidey-hole in her jaw, it flooded into her lymph nodes where they were currently fighting their own battle to rid it from her body.

Now she was fighting a battle too. With WBC numbers above 200 she felt that she *should* do chemo, but she just wasn't really *comfortable* with it. I told her that I'd look into treatments that might help in cleaning her lymph and blood and would get back to her in a few days.

The process I had in mind is called Photo-Oxidation and it uses ultraviolet (UV) light. Since nearly all bacteria may be killed or attenuated by UV rays I felt that it might do the trick of eliminating any "stuck" bacteria in her body no matter where it was hiding. Although many people look at Photo-Oxidation therapy as something very "new-agey", it isn't. Its use dates back to the 1940's pre-antibiotic days and had a cure rate of 98-100% in early and moderately advanced infections, and approximately 50% in terminally moribund patients. It fell out of vogue when the oh-so-convenient antibiotics made their appearances. Since there are far fewer practitioners out there still utilizing the technology, I really thought the hardest part would be finding someone she could get to. Strangely enough, there were not one but two practitioners about an hour away from where she lives.

When I made the call to give her the information on the practitioners I had located, she once again voiced her doubts. *Yes*, her WBC numbers are terrible. *Yes*, they need to come down. But chemo? It just didn't feel right to her. Again, I wrestled with what I *wanted* to say, and what I'm legally *allowed* to say. She really wanted my opinion and help, but I felt tongue tied.

Finally I made a strange request. I asked her to into her bathroom, which she did (all my clients should be so compliant). I told her to look, really look, at herself in the mirror. Then I asked her "Is that a sick woman"? A long silence. When she answered her voice was breaking "No Shauna. I don't see a sick woman."

Five days later, she called to tell me that she had changed her mind about doing chemotherapy at that time. She said that she just felt too good to be that sick, and had decided to trust her body instead of a test. She said "I just know what we're doing will work". She met with both of the UV light therapists and found one she liked. She said she laughed when she saw the questions asking about root canals and other dental work on her intake paperwork.

A few days ago I just happened to be standing next to the fax machine in my office when it started printing. I picked it up and looked at her new WBC number. 188.8, down from 202. I received an email from her the next day. I loved the last few lines; "Thanks for the referral to get the UV treatment. I can't wait to see what happens. Through this process I keep meeting more and more interesting people". I loved to hear that: Not calling it "cancer" anymore – now it was a "process"...

As of this writing, her numbers are continuing to fall, and although I can't yet know for certain since her case is ongoing, I feel confidant that they will continue their downward trend. After all, she's had that infection in her mouth for a long, long time, so I'm sure it will take some time to get the numbers all the way down to normal.

What I do know for sure is that even if her numbers go up and down a bit as her body continues to fight off the infection, it won't concern her so much. She knows in her heart that she's healthy. She can feel it in her body, and she's willing to trust her body over a test.

And what I also know is that the best part of her process for me was watching her go from a scared victim of a potentially deadly disease whose life was being ruled by "watching numbers" of the medical tests, to an empowered person making the calls that feel right to her. She got sick, and now she knows why. She's learned the lessons her dis-ease had to teach her, and it's time for it to go now. And I know that it will.

This book, or just this *chapter* for that matter, could be a thousand pages long. Just as I think I've seen it all (or most of it anyway) another oddball case comes through the door. Like the man who looked like a perfectly healthy guy until he took off his shirt and displayed a chest full of oozing wounds, the man whose skin just peeled off his hands one day (literally) like a glove for no particular reason, the 42-year-old woman who had had a tubal ligation who wanted me to help her get in shape to reverse it and hopefully get pregnant (her son is adorable), the woman with amoebic parasites in her knees causing her "arthritis" pain, and hundreds of others.

Maybe it sounds crazy to other people, but that's just a *day in the life* for a Naturopath worth her or his salt. I have always had a low threshold of boredom, so I guess I chose the right profession.

CHAPTER 9

The Mind and Healing

"It's supposed to be a secret, but I'll tell you anyway. We doctors do nothing. We can only help and encourage the doctor within."
— ALBERT SCHWEITZER, M.D.

Like it or not, I've found these statements are true in the vast majority of cases:

If you think you're going to get sick or stay sick – You will.

If you believe you are going to get well and stay well – You will.

If believe you won't or can't get well – You won't.

This may sound like an over-simplistic notion, but I'm telling you in my significant experience it's absolutely true. I have seen horribly ill, even "dying" people get well faster than you could possibly imagine, and many healthy or mildly ill people destroy themselves with their thoughts and obsessive worries or unconscious need to punish themselves. Some people do this subconsciously, and others on purpose. This is usually because they actually have an attachment or other somehow positive association with their illness, or sometimes because they are internalizing something from their past.

So what are "positive attachments" to illness? The most common one I see is attention. So few of us get the attention we feel we need and many people will either contrive an illness or hang on to one they no longer have so that they will finally get or sustain the attention they so desperately crave. Everyone – friends, family, strangers and especially spouses, all will pay attention to you, even wait on you if you're sick. For example, when a wife is chronically ill, you often hear from others that her husband "is so good to her". I've seen a lot of cases where although it is true now, he wasn't such a sweetie *before* she got sick.

And there are no special parking spaces for "well people" are there? Perhaps at the *back* of the parking lot?

The other most common one is leisure. If you are sick, you can't be expected to work, go to school or be otherwise productive. Instead, you are taken care of and/or pitied because you're "sick". I once saw a "chronically ill" teenager who finally admitted to me that if she got well, her parents would expect her to go to school or get a job. "Then what will happen to my art?" she asked.

The concept of "attachment to illness" was a very hard idea for me to understand and especially to accept as fact. Since I am the type of person who would stand on my head and eat Brussels sprouts (yuck) if it took me out of pain, it was incredibly tough to wrap my head around people who would purposefully and willfully stay sick. But after a few years in practice, I couldn't deny it any longer. I had just seen it too many times.

Most of us are guilty of this in small ways. As a kid you got "sick" the day of a test at school, or you are always "tired" in the morning on the days you have to go to the job you detest, but somehow you're feeling fine on the weekends. Or there's the frequent occurrence of someone having a "headache" when her partner is feeling inconveniently frisky. In the case of a lot of "A Type" personality adults this manifests in "breakdowns". Since these turbo-chargers won't give themselves permission to slow down or take days off, they become "ill" instead so that they have an excuse (mainly to themselves) where they are compelled to lay down and rest. These examples are relatively small and benign, very common and even understandable. Others however, can get pretty strange.

Once I suspect that a person is dealing with an attachment to an illness then the hardest part to figure out is; (a) Is he or she doing it consciously or subconsciously, and, (b) Can I talk to this person about it without him or her throwing something sharp at me? Attachment to illness can be very strong, and not everyone thanks me for bringing this potential to their attention.

A good example of the power of the subconscious connection was a woman in her early 30's who came in one day because of a horrible cough she'd been suffering with for years. Over the last several years she had been on dozens of different cough suppressants, allergy medications, asthma remedies, steroids and every kind of pill, puffer or shot known to medical science, all to no avail. When she came into my office she was currently taking six prescription medications for asthma, cough and allergies, and was still coughing every few seconds. I could even hear the poor thing hacking her brains out through the wall of my office while she was waiting for her appointment.

In addition to isodes and nosodes, the bio-resonant bio-feedback device I use also picks up emotional components since it deals with stress responses. I usually don't pay too much attention to this unless a particular emotion keeps repeating itself. In her case, the words "shame" and "guilt" popped up over and over. Time for tact. Very casually, and without looking directly at her, I asked, "Did you have a bit of a rough childhood?" Her response was immediate and dramatic. Looking exactly like the proverbial deer in the headlights, she said quietly "Why? Why would you say that?" I very matter-of-factly explained to her that my device was picking up the emotions of shame and guilt from her, and was reporting them as very important components in her symptomology. I told her that there was no need for her to tell me anything, I just wanted her to think about it and consider if those emotions could somehow be linked to her cough.

We were both quiet for a while (except for her coughing every few seconds) while she thought and I made notes, then she started to tell me her story. Her Father was a Vietnam vet who had suffered from Post-traumatic Stress Disorder. Her Mother had "had enough of it" and left her to "take care of him" when she was only eight years old. She tried as much as such a little girl possibly could, but always felt she was falling short. At her tender age, when other children were just getting around to *playing* house, she had total responsibility for everything in her house; cooking, cleaning, laundry and shopping. And just to make things worse, she feared and therefore avoided having any friends. She was terrified that if anyone was friendly with her and knew where she lived, that they may drop by some-time when her Father was out of control and yelling about "in-coming" and shoving her under the couch. She didn't think she could handle the embarrassment.

As she talked and talked on, I listened to her, but also kept a watchful eye on the clock behind her. I kept asking her ques-tions until enough time had passed that I was sure of what was happening. Finally, I asked her if she was aware that she had been talking about her Father and her childhood for a little over twenty minutes, and had not coughed *even once* during that pe-riod of time.

Her response was very unexpected. First she coughed then she jumped up from her chair, tearing off the electrical wrist-bands she was wearing while shouting at me, "You think I'm crazy? You're saying I'm crazy?" I tried to explain to her that in no way, shape or form did I think she was "crazy", I just thought that we had possibly discovered a component to her cough that maybe she hadn't considered before, and wasn't that great? She didn't think it was great at all! She remained very angry with me and left. Why would her emotions manifest as a cough? I have no idea. I only know that she quit coughing for over twenty minutes, apparently *for the first time in years,* while she was talking about her family. She never came back in again. I hope the little girl in her has quit coughing.

Another example of an unconscious connection was a very lovely woman who looked to be somewhere in her 50's, but turned out to be in her late 60's, and who came to see me about her puz-zling condition. She was a generally healthy person who took very good care of herself (hence the looking 10 years younger), and was great except for one annoying thing. She had a horrible itching skin rash over much of her body that just would not go away. Like many people who wind up in my office, she had tried "everything" over the last several years to no avail. The rash got less intense at times, but would then come roaring back with a vengeance.

The process of testing was puzzling too. At first I surmised that she was having the skin reaction from sugar, yet her sugar indicators were all fine. On questioning she revealed that she eats very little sugar, and was even more aware than most about the hidden sugars in foods. I thought perhaps, a sugar *allergy*? That would be really strange but not impossible, so over the next two months, we worked on some ways of desensitizing her system to sugar. This had some effect; the rash lessened, but it was still there. Weird.

On her third visit, she had just had a birthday. She told me that her rash was worse at the moment because her friend had given her a birthday present of some "incredibly decadent" chocolate and caramel turtles, and that she had been "horribly bad" and ate them all. The phrase "horribly bad" caught my attention. By the way, this lady is an accomplished psychotherapist and doesn't normally express that much judgment about herself or anyone else. I asked her why it was so "horribly bad" to enjoy a birthday present and she was momentarily stymied. She hadn't even realized she had used those particular words, and quickly recognized how out of character they were for her.

We decided to explore this thought, so I went to what I consider the obvious – her parents. I asked her what their attitude was toward sugar and junk food. She told me that her Mother was an adamant vegan who would not allow any sugar, sugared drinks or snacks in their home at all, ever. Laughing, she said that because of this prohibition, sugar became very desirable to her and she would "sneak it" at school. While her friends were doing drugs, she was doing Twinkies®! The look of "Aha" on her face after she said this was priceless.

From there, she used her incisive mind and therapeutic techniques on herself, and talked her way through it while I just listened. She had always felt guilty about sneaking the sugar, but her Mother punished her pretty severely whenever she got caught. Consequently she felt that although she would have an occasional transgression, she would always have to pay the piper so to speak. Therefore it was no coincidence that the rashes began shortly after the death of her Mother. Since her Mother was no longer there to catch and punish her for the sugar she still desired at times, she took on the job of punishment herself. Wow!

Following this realization, her rash cleared up almost immediately. It still amazes her (and me) that she can now eat sugar whenever she wants and it doesn't cause her any problem. As she explains it; she now lets her adult self be responsible for her healthy and limited sugar consumption, and has let go of the idea that she is "doing wrong" and needs to be punished. It's a good thing she's a therapist and gets this kind of thing. Most people get mad or look at me like I'm a loony if I suggest such a thing!

While these two examples obviously involve people who didn't know they were internalizing something, this third example is much more of a mystery for me. This woman in her early 40's told me she came to see me because her friends at church and her husband were "making her". This is my least favorite start, and as always when I hear these words, I told her she could leave if she wanted and I wouldn't tell on her. She decided to stay, but said "There probably won't be anything you can do for me." My second-least favorite start. This was not going well, and she'd only been in my office for five minutes.

Her symptoms were multiple and massive when combined. Out of 18 health questions on my intake form she had checked 13 of them as issues. She was always very tired, achy, depressed and nauseated, and couldn't lose any weight "no matter what she did", and despite being allergic to, in her words "all foods", she was well over 200 pounds, which made that a bit tough for me to believe. Obviously she was eating something! It's amazing how many times I've heard from people that they are "allergic" or otherwise sensitive to foods that are healthy, and that the "only thing they can hold down" is junk food. Very convenient if you ask me. And it makes absolutely no physiological sense.

These symptoms kept her not only from having a job, but from doing anything around the house like cooking, cleaning, shopping or laundry, as the minute she tried she got "too tired or nauseated". Her husband came home from work, fed the kids, cleaned the house and did laundry while she laid on the couch "too sick" to help. She said she'd been to every Allopathic doctor in the area and had been diagnosed with everything from Diabetes to Lupus to Fibromyalgia, but that no one had been able to do anything to make her feel any better. So she went to a well-known homeopathic doctor in Arizona. She showed me a huge fishing tackle box completely filled with the homeopathic remedies he had given her. As she informed me that "none of them worked". I noticed that most of the bottles were still half or more full. Hmmm.

Even though the red flags were now flapping manically in my head, I did a consultation with her anyway (I was in my second year and still naive). I didn't find anything too extreme health-wise, but I felt she would do well with a basic detox program. I suggested some supplements, made dietary changes, told her what kind of exercise to do, and sent her on her way.

A month later she returned. Before I could ask how she was doing, or could even sit down, she snapped, "Everything is worse than before! Nothing is better!" Okay. Did she take her supplements? "No", she responded, because they "made her sick". She based this on "feeling bad" when she took the very first dose, and never tried any of them again. Wasn't she already sick and feeling bad? No answer. Did she follow the dietary recommendations I made? No, because she "hates all those foods" I'd asked her to eat, and that was *a lot* of foods to hate. Did she get out and walk or otherwise exercise at all as I suggested? No, because she was "too tired, depressed and in pain" to move. I asked her how she expected anything to be different if she didn't do *any* of the things I suggested, or make any changes whatsoever. She seemed to understand that, and said she would make a better effort in the coming month.

As her next appointment day approached, a woman who went to church with her who is also a client of mine (and one of those who referred her to me), approached me in a health food store and told me how much better this other woman was doing. She said that this woman was out working with everyone else on the new church they were building, and she'd seen her shopping at a furniture store recently – things she never had the energy to do in the past. All right! Progress.

Then the woman came in for her appointment. She told me that even though she'd taken all the supplements exactly as I had said, she was feeling no better at all. Now first of all, I knew this was not a true statement. If she had indeed taken all the supplements as recommended, she would have had to buy more of one or two of them in order to last a full month, and a quick look in her chart told me she had not. I swear, I think people forget that I can count sometimes! At least she was honest enough to admit that she still "couldn't handle" the diet when I asked about that portion of the program.

I asked her about working at her church and furniture shopping and she got very quiet. She asked how I knew about that, and I told her. Her friend was happy for her and had told me. She then grudgingly relented that she had a "few moments" where she'd felt okay, but that was it. The rest of the time she was totally miserable.

At this point, I asked her kindly but straight out if she had any interest in getting well. She did not do what I recommended, would not admit that she ever felt better and yet kept coming back. So why come back? She got very indignant with me. Of course she wanted to get well; why wouldn't she? Well, you got me. I couldn't imagine why someone wouldn't want to feel better. So I gave her another opportunity, but told her that unless she worked *with* me to get well – *including the diet* – that I had no idea how to help her and there was no point in her continuing to see me. Naturopathy is lifestyle medicine, remember?

She came in a month later. She had not taken the supplements, worked on the diet or gotten any exercise. I very gently (and hopefully) professionally told her that I didn't think we were a good match. That I didn't want her wasting her time and money with me, and that she needed to see someone whom she trusted and would therefore do as he or she recommended. I told her that if she ever decided to actually try what I suggested that she was welcome to come back in, but without her participation there was nothing I could do. I also told her that in my mind, I felt that she could have an attachment to her illness and was unable to let it go. She told me I was heartless and didn't care about people, and left.

A few months later, I saw the friend of hers who had told me about her work and shopping expeditions. She had a different take on the whole situation. Apparently the woman's feeling a bit better had caused quite a problem in her life. When her husband saw her working at the church, he was ecstatic! He was so happy that she was off the couch, that he made the comment "If you keep getting well, you could even go back to work again." Oops. And when she was able to move around a bit, the people in her church weren't quite so willing to do absolutely everything for her. Double oops. No wonder she went back to being sick.

There is an interesting footnote to this. It was apparently not enough for this woman to just stop seeing me. She also told a dazzling array of very imaginative stories to her fellow church-goers who sent her in the first place. These tall tales ranged from the simple one: That I couldn't figure out what was wrong with her and I had "broken down crying" telling her that she was "out of my league", to a very involved and vague story where I was apparently "just about to be arrested for something". Whenever anyone asked what I was allegedly being arrested for, she said she "wasn't allowed to tell". Allowed by whom? Apparently that was also a secret. I was constantly being told a new story by various amused folks who knew her. Oh yes, just for the record, I have never broken down crying in front of a client, thought one was "out of my league" or been arrested "for something".

So, which was it? Was she attached to her illness in a subconscious or conscious way? Was she unaware of her motivations, or was she using her "illness" so that she didn't have to work or take care of her house? Did the thought that everyone she knew would quit asking constantly about her health and stop assuring her over and over that they were "praying for her" if she felt better send her over the edge? I have no idea. Although I have had many people with very odd attachments to their illness since then, this one still stands out in my mind as the most extreme and puzzling.

Another manifestation of the mind/body connection relates to the heavily discussed "placebo effect". Very often when a person is healed by natural means, it is written off dismissively as being from a "placebo effect", essentially saying that the person so believed that he or she was going to get well, it happened. So where's the problem with that? In my mind, if a person gets well, then excellent! Fantastic! I could care less what made them well as long as they *get* well. And what better way to get well than by tapping the limitless power of your own positive mind?

As I've mentioned previously, Naturopaths are not allowed to utter words like "cure", "treat", "heal" or even "help". It's hard to give someone hope without using any of these words, but somehow we find a way. Giving hope to the hopeless is a large part of what I and most Naturopaths do. I can never make promises to anyone as to the outcome, but I *can* promise to do my best to help. This alone is all a lot of people need to hear. Just having someone willing to try is often a boost.

There is however, a flip side to this. A dark side that I have not often heard discussed, especially in the allopathic community. If your mind is acknowledged to be so powerful that it is able to heal you of symptoms, than must not the converse be true that the mind is also powerful enough to kill you? When someone is told by his or her doctor, "You've got six weeks to live", "You're going to have this disease for the rest of your life", or "There's nothing that can be done for your pain", isn't this doctor then contributing to killing the patient's hope, and possibly, his or her body?

If Allopaths can condemn natural practitioners by saying that our treatments did nothing, that it was just the client's expectation and hope that made him or her well, then isn't the reverse also true? By telling people they're going to be sick or in pain forever, or that they will die soon, aren't you planting *that* thought into their minds so strongly that it can actually help it to occur? If you believe one potential, then don't you have to believe the other?

How many times have you heard someone say, "The doctor said aunt Marge had three months to live, and she died three months later almost to the day. Can you believe that?" Yes, I can! I've seen people so convinced that they were going to die, that there is no power in heaven or on earth that could talk them out of it. What makes anyone think that he or she can plant these "hopeless" ideas in people's minds, and then expect them to have a serious shot at any better outcome?

Two different women I saw several years apart are prime examples of this concept. They had a lot in common: They were both right around 50, they both had cancer (one ovarian, one breast), and they had both been told they probably only had "3 to 6 weeks to live" by their doctors. However, they had one huge difference: Attitude. One of these ladies, no matter how much better she got, continued to act as if she was sick. Her life was a round of special foods, doctor's appointments, physical therapies, naps, and going to the hospital emergency room for everything, even simple things like a day of diarrhea. A year and a half after first being told she had "3 to 6 weeks to live" she was still behaving like an invalid.

To the complete contrary, the other woman never behaved a single day as if she was ill. When I started with the obligatory legal stuff about conventional cancer treatment, she impatiently waved her hand at me to stop. "I know that legally you can't suggest that I say no to chemo, but *I* can. It's my body and I say 'No!' So don't waste my time on that, okay?" Okay lady, you're the boss! She jumped on all the information I gave her like the proverbial duck on a June bug, and dug in as if her life depended on it – which she felt it did. It's too bad that people often have to get this sick in order to change their lifestyles, but my goodness this woman was perfect. Enough water, right foods, exercise, supplements right on time, everything.

She came in after her first month raring to go for more. When I asked how she was doing, she leaned forward onto my desk and said "I feel great. What are we going to do now?" with an expectant smile. After giving her the recommendations on supplements for the next month, I gave her something else that

I've told several others that I thought she needed. It's not every-one who I could impart this kind of advice to, but I felt I could with her.

Prefacing it by telling her I knew it might sound crazy, I told her that I felt she needed to find a way, truly in her heart, to find gratitude that she got cancer. As I knew she would, she looked at me like I was crazy, but she also said she'd give it some thought as I hadn't steered her wrong yet. She called several weeks later to give me some news. First, after looking at what positive changes had been made, not only in her but in her entire family as a result of the healthier lifestyle she had embraced, she'd found a way to be grateful for getting cancer. Because of the dietary and other changes, not only was she feeling great, but her husband had lost twenty pounds, her kids had lost many little health issues that had been plaguing them, and her brother was no longer a "borderline diabetic". She felt that if she hadn't had cancer she and her family would still be trudging along with all their old, unhealthy bad habits, and her whole family had now made a new start on healthier lives. After hearing this, I wasn't as surprised by her second piece of news: Her tumor had now shrunk from "the size of a golf ball to the size of a quarter" in this short time.

Obviously the supplements and her lifestyle changes were making a big difference, but the biggest change, and the one I think truly was healing her, was taking place in her mind and her heart. To her, she wasn't sick now and because of her new lifestyle, she never would be sick again, and she was truly grate-ful for the lesson this cruel invader of her body had taught her. There is no doubt in my mind that this amazing lady was heal-ing herself with her strong positive attitude and her grateful and giving heart. She is truly an inspiration.

But having said that, there are some people who just don't want to believe in the power of the mind. There have been a few feeble attempts to actually sue Naturopaths and other natu-ral practitioners for "giving false hope" to someone. It's impor-tant to note that these legal cases are usually brought about by another member of the family who doesn't believe in natural medicine, and/or doesn't think that the loved one is capable of making his or her own rational choices. That rather than being believers and following their own hearts and minds, they have been "bamboozled" by someone just trying to make a buck off them.

These cases are *rarely* brought by the person being treated. Admittedly there are more than a few snake-oil salesmen out there robbing people, but there are also countless more who are just willing to help a hopeless person find some hope. Not promises, just an offer of help. And FYI, if you're just trying to fleece people of money, I'll bet there are a lot easier ways to accomplish that than being a Naturopath that does business by referrals; trust me on this one!

So ask yourself this: When was the last time an Allopath was dragged into court because they gave false *negative* expectations? A number of people who see me were told they would never recover or were about to die, but they get well instead. And none of them to my knowledge has ever sued the doctor for giving him or her false *negative* expectations. While I understand that a lot of these doctors are trying to not give false hope to someone they honestly believe won't recover, or maybe just in efforts to not get sued, it seems to me that they are implanting a lot of negative expectation.

Since I'm talking about the mental effect on healing, an uncomfortable word needs to be said here, not to those who are suffering from illness, but to the families and loved ones of these people. Although it may be hard for loved ones to understand, I have found in my personal experience that you can't force anyone to get well. There are many people out there who know exactly what it will take for them to be well, and they make the conscious decision *to not do it*. And there is nothing anyone else can do to change their minds. This spans the gamut from simply keeping their symptoms as is, having to take prescription drugs with awful side effects, having surgeries they could have avoided, and yes, even *dying* when they know just what could have been done to avoid it.

As hard as it is for me to understand that a person would rather die than give up a particular lifestyle choice or even a *particular food*, I have seen it more than once. This is especially common among diabetics, but I've seen it in multiple other situations as well. Many of these people have told me straight out that they know for a fact if they just started (or stopped) doing a particular thing, like starting to exercise or stopping eating so much sugar or grains, they would be well, but they make the choice to not do so. And once someone has made this choice, there is very little chance that the begging and pleading of someone who cares about them will do much good. So my (admittedly tough) advice to loved ones, hard as it is, is to give it up and accept such a choice.

It is not uncommon for a grieving person (usually the husband or wife, sometimes another relative) to either call or come in and tearfully beg me to get the sick person "to listen to reason" and to try to survive. I got one of these calls very recently from a husband who desperately wants his wife to get involved in her care. Her doctor told her that "no matter what you do, you're going to die sometime between two weeks and two months, so you may as well enjoy yourself." He advised her to "have chocolate shakes everyday, eat whatever you want, do whatever you want" because she was going to die anyway, and this man's wife wanted to do just that – keep all the habits that got her sick in the first place, and die on the doctor's schedule. What I told the husband, as I've told so many others, is that *this is her choice, not yours*. Try to accept her choice. Since originally seeing her I had received multiple phone calls from him and his daughter, and not one from the client herself. Her choice seemed very clear to me.

He was also angry about his perception that the other doctor was "giving up on her". I tried to tell him that the other doctor was only going on what he thought was right. He honestly felt in his heart and by virtue of his education and experience that there was no chance of saving her so she might as well enjoy what was left of her life, so to him that was a kind choice. I say this over and over to people: As health care workers, we all do what we think is right; *that's why we do it*! Her MD thinks it's right to make the end of people's lives as easy as possible; I choose to help those people who are not ready to go, to hang in there. That's what we both feel is right, which is why we practice as we do.

Many seem to like to think of natural healers as "charlatans" who take advantage of sick people by giving them false hope. I prefer to think of it as not giving up on someone who still has fight left in them. If someone is ready to die, than that's his or her decision and everyone around this person should try to accept it. But if one wants to keep trying, why give up on him or her? Why not help such a person to the best of my abilities? I don't always win with these people, but they are always happy with their decisions. Even if they ultimately lose their battle with life, they go out feeling good, in charge, and still swinging.

In any case, I would much rather be the one planting the idea of hope and recovery in a person than the one seeding his or her mind with thoughts of endless illness or death. Hope, as tenuous as it can be, is never "false" to me.

CHAPTER 10

The War on "Which" Drugs?

"The whole imposing edifice of modern medicine, for all its breath-taking successes, is, like the celebrated Tower of Pisa, slightly off balance. It is frightening how dependant on drugs we are all becoming and how easy it is for doctors to prescribe them as the universal panacea for all our ills."

— HRH PRINCE CHARLES, PRINCE OF WALES

"The War on Drugs" is a statement I'm almost as tired of hearing as "The War on Cancer". Does anyone recall which U.S. President officially started "The War on Cancer"? I'll remind you. One Richard Millhouse Nixon, President of the United States between 1969 and 1974. And since that time, despite billions and billions of dollars flushed down the toilet of "research" every year, we are drowning in a cancer rate that gets worse every year. And don't fool yourself. We're drowning in drugs too.

Oh no, not just the ones from Colombian drug lords, but rather the ones flung at you from every angle and for every conceivable thing in life at an ever-increasing rate by aggressive advertising campaigns and your local trusty Dr. Feelgood. You can now take a prescription pill for "chronic dry eye", for "restless legs", or for improving "bladder control". And young women are lining up in droves so that they don't have to be inconvenienced by monthly menstruation; as a birth control pill now can stop this natural function almost completely!

When I was a kid, MAD Magazine did a spoof on the TV show "Marcus Welby, MD" (about the life and times of a kindly doctor) and called it "Makeus Sickby, MD." I used to think that was funny. But the sad fact is, according to newest statistics, you might be able to get into a lot more danger through your local doctor's office than your random Colombian drug lord, and the docs are a lot more accessible. After all, you'll rarely find a Colombian drug lord listed in the local Yellow Pages.

As a rule, I am very close-mouthed with clients about my personal life. Despite this desire for privacy on my part, people often try to figure out my political affiliations for whatever reasons of their own, so I will say this now on the subject of politics and Presidents. Whoever starts caring about this crisis of prescription drugs and iatrogenic deaths in this country and will work to change that situation, I will vote for he, she or it no matter what party ticket that individual is running on or what planet he, she or it hails from. And please make it soon. Enough said.

You could say that I come by my distaste for prescription drugs naturally since my parents weren't big on them either. My brother and I didn't receive vaccines and since our family doctor was a chiropractor, we didn't take antibiotics or other drugs either. Although my brother and I rarely got sick, my Mother had a very specific prescription for the cold/flu/sore throat kind of thing: Chicken noodle or tomato soup with crackers, grape juice, and bed rest with a favorite story read to us, and let me tell you, it was very effective. And like the Father character in "My Big Fat Greek Wedding" who thought that Windex® cured everything, my Father also had a "drug of choice": Campho-Phenique®. Whatever was wrong in your system, my Dad was absolutely convinced that all that was needed was a little Campho-Phenique®, and it's amazing how often he was right. Other "cure-all" choices in my family include Castor Oil from my grandmother, and Absorbine Jr.® from my uncle, so I guess the fact that prescription drugs are anathema to me should come as no big surprise.

The *Journal of the American Medical Association* (JAMA) prints a lot of statistics. A recent report names "The Top Three Causes of Unnecessary Deaths in the United States" and it's very scary. Actually, the title itself makes me wonder: If this addresses "unnecessary" deaths, what exactly would be categorized as "necessary" deaths? Anyway, I digress... so what would *your* first guess be? I asked a lot of people and they mostly said "Cancer". A good guess, since it seems everyone has it nowadays, but nope. Cancer is actually the number three killer on the hit parade. Heart Disease would be a better guess, since it comes in at number two.

Number one however, is the aforementioned "iatrogenic" deaths. According to my dictionary of medical terms, "iatrogenic" is defined as "pertaining to a condition caused by medical diagnostic procedures, or exposure to medical treatment, facilities and personnel." In other words, a doctor, a procedure, a prescription drug or a hospital staff member caused the *death*. Not injury or illness, but unnecessary, avoidable death. Your friendly local Marcus Welby and his buddy Big Pharma together represent the top leading cause of unnecessary death in the United States. *That*, my friends, is crazy!

Toxic Cocktails

By far, the most common cause of iatrogenic death is an adverse reaction to prescription drugs. Although studies vary a bit, the number of deaths **reported** in the U. S alone is estimated to be between 44,000 (that's the *low* number) and 106,000 people each and every year – *just* from drugs used as prescribed by their doctors. Even using the low number (if you can call 44,000 deaths "low"), that's still more people killed annually by legal prescription drugs than by breast cancer, AIDS, or car accidents. And here we were worried about Swine Flu!

Now if you add in the death toll being attributed to medical error, unnecessary procedures, hospital infections and other "iatrogenic" identified causes, then we're looking at an unfathomable total of well over 780,000 people per year, in the U.S. alone (you can locate these and other such disturbing statistics by Internet searching for "Table of Iatrogenic Deaths in the United States").

To put that gruesome statistic into some relatable context, let me give you a visual that I often give people in seminars: If eight 250-passenger jumbo jets collided in mid-air and killed everyone aboard all planes (that's about 2,000 people), you'd hear about it on the news in darkest Africa! Yet that number is about equivalent to how many people die of iatrogenic causes **each and every day in the U.S. alone**. Why is one statistic quickly recognized for the human "tragedy" that it is, and the other discarded and ignored?

The statistics of medical-related deaths are really sickening (pun intended) any way you look at it – the number-one cause of death in America! 9/11 was a terrible tragedy where nearly three thousand people lost their lives, but there are other casualties to think about as well. Keep in mind that over the ten years following 9/11, more than 7 million Americans have <u>died</u> from the unintentional consequences of their FDA-approved, doctor-prescribed drugs, combined with the inadvertent mistakes of physicians, surgeons, medical treatments or diagnostic procedures.*

This was the statistic as of the time I was writing this book. Unfortunately it may be staggeringly higher by the time you actually read this.

As crazy as this all is, unfortunately it doesn't surprise me. After all, I'm a Naturopath, so a sizeable portion of those I see as clients are "ones that got away" – the people hideously damaged "iatrogenically", but not quite dead. And as Billy Crystal said in "The Princess Bride", "Mostly dead, is not dead." So off we go in attempting to somehow repair the damage done.

Honestly, the way drugs are layered on and combined with people, I'm frankly surprised that there aren't even *more* deaths. I recently saw a man in his late 70's who was on *17 prescriptions*; among them were three heavy hitter anti-depressants (note: He was only *depressed* about being *sick*!), two blood thinners, two heart medications, five blood pressure pills, and just in case his liver wasn't chewed up enough by the drugs, a statin cholesterol medication. According to the PDR, there were at least five known contraindications among these drugs, meaning that they shouldn't be taken together according to accepted medical science. The heart medications had brought his heart rate down so low that his doctor had *installed a pacemaker* to bring it back up again!

I silently wondered why they didn't just take him off one of the meds, but hey, I'm just a Naturopath and have to be very careful what I say that may sound like "criticism" of a doctor, so instead I clenched my teeth (some more) and let him continue his story. When his stomach got upset *on his 17 medications* (go figure), his doctor took his gallbladder out! It didn't help, and now he can't digest fats to boot, so they upped his cholesterol drug. And do you know what his question was – why he actually came to see me? He wanted to know why he is so tired all the time and also impotent. I wanted to know why he was upright and not dead! By the way, this man was referred to me by a pharmacist who is one of my many "closet clients".

One of the many things I find a constant puzzlement is how easily people will take prescription drugs with no questions asked. Heaven knows they don't do that with natural stuff! Ironic, ain't it? Most people want to know exactly what everything I suggest for them is for, how it works and if there will be any potential side effects from every single natural substance I give them.

That's fine with me, and in fact I'm glad they ask, but I find it an unusual dichotomy that they will take, let's say, Coumadin®, which is Warfarin sodium (Warfarin being the active ingredient in *rat poison*) with no question or hesitation, but want to know if the asparagus juice they will be taking is going to cause any problems! By the way, if you don't believe me on the rat poison thing, just look at the PDR or packet insert on Coumadin®, then take a peek at the rat poison box in your local hardware store, and you will see the exact same ingredient listed – Warfarin sodium. And, if you still don't believe me, just check the website www.rxlist. com and read the blaring warning, and I quote: "Warfarin sodium can cause major or fatal bleeding." And I don't know about you, but this thought strikes me as odd: If a drug needs to be tested for effectiveness and safety, they test it on lab rats, right? So when tested on rats, Warfarin *kills* them, but it is somehow still considered acceptable for use in humans. So what exactly are they testing for?

When a new client comes in I always ask for a list of his or her prescription drugs and supplements so that I can make sure nothing I want to suggest will contraindicate with anything already being taken. Not that there are many contraindications with herbals, but there are a few, and I'm very careful about them. Just as a couple of examples, I don't recommend taking potassium supplements along with some blood pressure meds, and there is a wide variety of food supplements, herbs and enzymes that are not suggested for use along with the aforementioned Coumadin® (heaven forbid that an herbal causes problems with the effectiveness of their rat poison!).

Although most folks are taking "the usual suspects" of drugs that I have grown accustomed to seeing, sometimes I see one I don't understand or don't recognize, so I ask the client what it's for. When I ask this, more often than I would think even possible, I hear "I don't know." In other words, these people are putting at best, unnatural chemicals, and at worst, poisons, into their bodies and they have absolutely no idea *why*. I have seen any number of very pale faces when I print out a PDR or Rxlist report for them and they realize that they're on drugs they don't have any idea why they'd be taking them, and/or see those with frightening side effects and poor track records. Mind you, these are not printouts from some whacko Naturopathic counter-information source, these are straight from Physicians' Desk Reference (PDR), the very same source given out free to every MD and pharmacy in the country.

The Big Business of Depression

The most common occurrence is talking with people who have no idea that they are on one or more anti-depressants. They come to me usually because of fatigue, weight gain, dry mouth, digestive problems and low libido, only to find out that they are on an anti-depressant that they don't even know why they are taking, and that their symptoms described above reads like a laundry list of the "acceptable side effects" of these drugs. It used to be that I would ask, "Why are you taking an anti-depressant?" when someone listed Paxil®, Zoloft®, Celexa®, Effexor®, Cymbalta® or Prozac®, but now I have learned to rephrase my question as: "So what is the (insert above anti-depressant brand here) for?" because they often don't even know that they're taking an anti-depressant.

Asked the first way, I got a lot of "WHAT? What are you talking about?" reactions. Asked the second way, I get some very strange answers indeed ranging from the legitimate reason of depression to (according to medical journals) some very iffy indications, to flat out lies. One woman told me that her doctor told her that the Zoloft® was for her "exocrine system". My next question to her was "Do you know what your exocrine system does?" She didn't, so I explained it. I'm very glad I'm not that doctor – she was pretty upset.

Anti-depressants are a very mixed bag to me anyway. Prescriptions for anti-depressants were relatively rare prior to the mid-1980's, reaching a previously unseen high of 2.5 million prescriptions per month by 1988. This seems like a whopper of an increase over such a short period of time, even if you do take into account the understandable depression caused by disco music. But from there it just didn't slow down. By 2010 there were more than 12 million anti-depressant prescriptions being filled *per month* in the U.S. alone, and the increase in anti-anxiety drugs (like Xanex®) for 10 to 19 year olds went up full **50%** from 2000 to 2010. Wait a minute… 10 to 19 year olds? And here I thought anxiety was a natural part of being a teenager!

By 2005, 10 of the Top 100 most prescribed drugs were now anti-depressants, with Xanax® (an anti-anxiety drug) and Zoloft® (an SSRI, or selective serotonin reuptake inhibitor) at positions #9 and #16 respectively, and with Lexapro® (also an SSRI) hard on their heels at #17. Collectively in 2005, the Top 10 antidepressants had a total of 200,401,000 prescriptions written for the year, which represented nearly 17 million scripts every month (source: RxList.com).

And the "hit parade" continues. Prozac®, once the reigning king of anti-depressants, had dropped to a lowly #29 on the list.

Possibly because of the heavy duty warnings and Congressional hearings on the increased numbers of suicides (especially in kids and teens) while on the drug, or maybe just because they aren't doing the amount of television advertising that some of the others do. Paxil® (a "comer" at #38 with a bullet) and Wellbutrin XL (at #66) have done very well with their TV ads. Cymbalta®, a relative newcomer to the pack didn't quite make the Top 100 – it was at #101 in 2005, bringing in a mere 4,938,000 scripts written, but I'm sure they're doing much better all the time. Their ads are really good.

Just to give you an idea of how much money is spent on these drugs, the top-three anti-depressants that are all in the overall Top 20 "most prescribed drugs" are Xanax® (number 9 and the most expensive), Zoloft® (number 16 and the second most expensive of the three), and Lexapro® (number 17 and the least expensive of the three). These three drugs alone are raking in $11,336,458,000 a year. That's a lot of commas, so let me be very clear: That is 11 billion, 336 million, 458 thousand dollars, for just those three. This amount of money being spent combined with the commonly listed side effects of a 10-20 pound weight gain, gastrointestinal problems, loss of sex drive, and the ever-popular "increase in suicidal ideation" seems like enough to depress anyone. I really don't get the concept here: I'm depressed, so please let me gain a bunch of weight, lose my energy and my desire to have sex, and disengage my conscience and concern for others to the point that I can more easily commit suicide – that'll make me feel better! But despite that, depression my friends is big business.

How big that business really is, recently came to me in a very strange and creepy way. While driving in extremely heavy traffic in Santa Fe, New Mexico, I actually got nervous wondering how many of my bumper-to-bumper buddies were at this very moment driving in an altered state on their legally prescribed anti-depressants. Not a happy thought.

According to Drugs.com list of pharmaceutical sales for 2010, the trend for antidepressants continues, but with an alarming amount of anti-psychotic and ADD/ADHD drugs now making the

Top 100. Abilify®, a drug being now prescribed for Alzheimer's came in at #6. If you look up the side effects on this one… is it just me, or do they sound exactly like Alzheimer's?

Drugs with the SSRI classification (of which there are many) have built-in perpetuity so to speak. Once you start taking them, the pineal and pituitary glands that are responsible for secreting serotonin, become lazy over time and stop working, virtually guaranteeing that you will need the drug for life. Anti-depressants of course, are just the (more obvious and discussed) tip of the iceberg. There are also the pain killers such as Vioxx® that have now been taken off the market, but not before they contributed to the deaths of (depending on the particular re-port) no less than many thousands of people.

One last word on anti-depressants: If the much-beloved-by-Allopaths double-blind studies on drugs are really that im-portant, then why are anti-depressants *still* on the market? In JAMA's double-blind studies (most recently in Jan 2010) they stacked Zoloft® and Paxil® against placebos, and the placebos won! People actually felt better taking the placebos than the drugs! Apparently some double-blind studies are more impor-tant than others. I suppose if they could find a way to make pla-cebos prescription only, then…

Apparently a lot more "proof" of harm is necessary in the case of prescription drugs than with herbal supplements as the prescriptions have to kill people more on a scale with Pol Pot before they get yanked, and herbals go at the first hint of "suspicion". You've probably heard of Ephedra, an herb that is most commonly used (very effectively I might add) for asthma, allergies and bronchial conditions since it mimics the effects of adrenaline. While I fully admit that Naturopathic medicine has no place in emergency medicine (one of the many reasons I got into it – no 3:00am emergency calls for me, thank you) I used it to great benefit on myself when I had an anaphylactic response to a brown recluse spider bite and it almost instantly reopened my lungs.

However, as is the situation with most herbals, there are multiple applications and potential effectiveness for Ephedra.

Although not its primary use to herbalists, its secondary use as a metabolic stimulant became better known, which resulted in it popping up as an ingredient in all kinds of OTC (over the counter) diet and "pep" pills. While it is true that this is one of the few herbals that does have some contraindications (*i.e.* don't use it if you have high blood pressure, an overactive thyroid, diabetes or insomnia), those contraindications were clearly listed on the product labels, and there were always suggested dosages listed for the product. Ephedra was pulled from the market (although it has now been reinstated) because it was "suspected" as a "possible contributing factor" in five deaths. Notice the words "suspected", "possible" and "five". Compare this to what it took for Vioxx®, Thalidomide or dozens of other such "FDA approved" prescription drugs to get the big yank.

One of the reasons that the temporary ban on Ephedra was overturned was because when these deaths were investigated, it was found that the people in question had taken a *500% to 600% overdose* of the suggested dosage. Think about it for a moment: If the doctor gave you a drug and the suggested dosage was one pill, and you took five or six of them at a time and died, would anyone blame the *drug*? No way! They'd blame the dummy who took the overdose! So why is this accusatory finger pointed so quickly at a supplement, and so slowly (dare I say, arthritically?) at a prescription drug?

In 2007 I stopped purchasing future hard copies of the PDR, but I did keep 2002 and 2007 copies of the PDR for "Nonprescription Drugs, Dietary Supplements and Herbs" on my bookshelf. I now use the online version of the PDR for a couple of reasons: First, new drugs are added far faster than the books can be printed and I often need to look up something a client is taking that it is "too new" for the publication date, and second, these weighty and expensive things take up a ridiculous amount of shelf space since they are about seven inches wide and weigh about nine pounds!

The PDR for prescription applications is exclusively that, prescription drugs only, with nothing else included. The one for the non-prescription applications on the other hand, not only includes natural substances like herbals and nutraceuticals, but also a huge host of *un*-natural products like OTC medications for pain, colds and yeast infections, plus vitamins manufactured by pharmaceutical companies that are so full of toxins and chemicals that no Naturopath would ever suggest anyone use them. In fact, there are very few pages in this book dealing with anything a Naturopath would work with, but despite that fact it is still only 841 pages long. The 2002 drug PDR on the other hand is 3,635 pages long, and could crush a small child. I shudder to think what the most current version looks like.

I thought long and hard about how much I wanted to say about specific prescription drugs, and came to two conclusions: (1) I could easily write a whole book on the world of the pharmaceutical industry and the poison it dishes out, and (2) there already exists a whole library of such books and websites out there. Entire books (many of them, and written by both Allopathic and Naturopathic doctors) have been published about subjects such as the sickening and disastrous results of over-prescribing antibiotics; not the least of which is the current strains of "smart bugs" that have mutated to the point that drugs are ineffective.

At a global conference on integrative medicine I attended, I listened (in awe) to a gastroenterologist who was asking his Allopathic colleagues to "face facts" and realize that there were many conditions (he cited both Metabolic Syndrome X that affects about 70 million Americans, and the far too common Staph infection as only two of them) that drugs "cannot touch". He encouraged them all to seek out something that would, and actually suggested taking Traditional Naturopaths, people specifically trained in the use of herbals and other non-drugs, into their practices as respected colleagues! Too bad so few seem to agree with him.

To be sure, I could write copious pages about the usurious and immoral markup on drugs, about the damage they cause (often the listed side effects are worse than the disease), about the fact that drug ads admonish you to "Tell your doctor if you have liver disease" (aren't *they* supposed to tell *you* that?), about the cascade that begins once you step on the drug merry-go-round and the side effects of one drug leads to the need for another, and another, and so on. As an example; taking a leading thyroid medication leads to bone loss, which necessitates that you take drugs for that, which cause acid reflux so you take an acid inhibitor, which leads to... you get the point. Is it any surprise at all that there are literally billions of prescriptions filled every year in America alone? Are *you* taking 6, 10, 12 drugs? Speaking for myself, my family and most of my clients; we're not on *any*, so someone is making up for ours! I sure hope it's not you!

And on that topic, it amazes me how often people ask me if I think antibiotics and other specific drugs are "okay" to take. As stated before, it is against the law for me to advise anyone not to take a prescribed drug, so that must be my consistent response to them. But think for a moment, people – I'm a *Naturopath*! What do you *think* I think of these poisonous substances? Duh!

Then we come to diagnostic testing and other "routine" procedures. Many people will never have to worry about the diseases and conditions for which they are getting routinely tested, since the tests themselves have the capability of getting them before a disease does! Understand this simple fact: *Scientists agree that there is no safe dose for radiation*. They have come up with the term "acceptable", but there is no such thing as *safe*. And the RAD's (which is defined as "a dosage of absorbed radiation") emitted particularly by a mammogram, something considered "routine", are exceptionally high.

A 1995 study by Dr. John Gofman estimated that "three-quarters of the current annual incidence of breast cancer in the United States is being caused by earlier ionizing radiation, primarily from medical sources." The eminent researcher Dr. Irwin Bross came to the same conclusion (in the 1970's) regarding leukemia, citing that the massive increase in the disease was primarily caused from medical radiation. Interestingly enough, Dr. Bross had been hired and his research funded by none other than the National Cancer Institute to find out why leukemia rates were skyrocketing. The folks there didn't care much for his conclusions and not surprisingly, cut off his funding!

When looking at doing "routine" testing, you also have to contemplate what you would do with your test results. I often ask people what they plan on doing with the results, which I think is a reasonable question. If you decide to go the Naturopathic direction to address even the *slightest* negative test result, just know that you may be in for a battle. One of my clients who decided to go the natural route with her breast cancer found it necessary to go to a doctor other than the one who gave her the diagnosis in order to track her progress. When she decided to make her own call and take what she thought in her heart was the right path, her oncologist stopped returning her phone calls. Her new doctor honored her decision and is thrilled with her rapid progress, but not everyone gets that lucky with their doctors.

So I guess my "last words" on drugs or on any medical procedure is THINK FIRST. Don't take a drug without knowing what it's for and what the possible side effects are. Go to the PDR or Rxlist website, or just get out a magnifying glass and read the dang insert folded into the pill box, but don't go in blind! When you were a little kid, you were told to "Stop, Look and Listen" before crossing the street. I'm saying to you now to "Stop, Look and Listen" before you ingest any unnatural substance, or let someone cut, poison or burn you. NEVER have to respond "I don't know" when someone asks why you've had a vital organ removed!

Sometimes you'll still decide to do it, but please, know *why* first. Stop: Slow down and think. Look: Do your own research. The Internet makes that a lot easier. Listen: Ask questions! And most important: Never, *never* forget that it's *your* body, and therefore *your* choice. People often say to me that their doctor is "making them" take a drug or do a procedure, and this is not the case (at least not yet). *As hard as they may try to make you believe it, no one can make you do something you don't want to do to your own body.* So stop using them as your excuse.

It's up to you to make the right choices, so grab the reins and make them! As a friend of mine says, buck up there, cowboy!

CHAPTER 11

Vaccines: What's Really in Them, and Your Legal Rights

"Why would a patient swallow a poison because he is ill, or take that which would make a well man sick?"

— L.F. KEBLER, M.D.

This was a really difficult chapter to write, and in fact, I wrote it last. There is so much controversy and question surrounding vaccines and I get so crazy over the injustice of it that it makes it a most challenging subject for me to tackle. My staff could tell when I was working on this and would inform people, "It's not a good time to talk to her; she's researching vaccines." Man this stuff gets to me!

Keep in mind when reading this that this is *my* book, and therefore contains *my* formed opinions and *my* experiences. I invite you to do your own research and make your own choice. A really good place to start on this is at www.nvic.org (the National Vaccine Information Center), and while you're there please consider giving all the support and money you can to the very brilliant and hard-working Barbara Loe Fisher and team. Her Center has excellent and up-to-date information and is truly fighting on the front line of this ugly battle to inform the public about potential dangers involving vaccines.

As I've said, my parents (thank you, thank you) decided against vaccines for me, and I feel as if I've dodged a lot of bullets that other people my age struggle with as a result of it. For the record, my personal and continuing choice is that I don't do Allopathic vaccines of any kind myself.

I decided that the way to start this chapter is to simply inform or remind you of your rights (such as they are) concerning vaccines. Most people assume they are absolutely mandatory, and schools and other governmental agencies definitely reinforce that false notion. Truth is; they aren't totally. Different States have different regulations (see NVIC's map for the particular and most current State exemptions), but in every State in the union there is some *legitimate exemption from vaccines if you choose to use it*. There are three primary accepted exemptions:

1. **Medical**: There is some medical reason for being exempt, for example, you or your child are already sick or immune compromised, or have shown previous reactivity to vaccines. **This one will apply in every State**.
2. **Religious**: Seems clear enough – you object on religious grounds. Several organized religions object to either any or undue medical intervention. I don't have to name the religions since I'm sure you know if yours is one of them or not! **This one applies everywhere except Mississippi and West Virginia.**
3. **Philosophical:** What does that mean? It means that simply as a thinking human being, you have decided against vaccinations. As of this writing, this exemption is available in quite a few States, including Colorado, where I live and currently practice.

Are these easy to assert? Well, not easy, but if you don't want vaccines for your family, then it's worth the time. The medical exemption has to be accompanied by a letter from a licensed physician stating that the physical condition of the person is such that the immunization could endanger their health or life. This can be a bit tough as most "licensed physicians" see no problem with vaccines and there are currently no processes being used to screen out children who may be vulnerable. However, if you have a doctor willing to work with you, this one is probably the best. And that, in and of itself, seems odd to me. With all the research being done with other diseases that only affect a finite amount of the populace, there is *no* study being done to determine the long-term effects of vaccines – something that both the greater medical community and the government wants everyone to take no matter what. Why?

The religious exemption is a little easier, as you do it yourself. You submit a form to the school (or other that wants you to get the vaccines) saying that the parent or guardian of a minor (an "emancipated minor" or adult would do this for themselves) is opposed to immunizations because they are "adherent to a religious belief whose teachings are opposed to immunizations". Thank goodness you don't need a letter from anyone on this one. Who would you get it from anyway? Now *that* could take some doing!

The philosophical exemption doesn't require much to be written, but from my research it looks like you follow the same general procedure as with the religious one – declare in writing that you have a "personal belief that is opposed to immunizations". Maybe you can describe your personal belief such as, "I don't care to have live virus, toxic metals, a flotsam and jetsam of gooey tissue ingredients and other harmful chemicals injected into me", or "I'd rather not take any increased chance of my child becoming autistic, thank you". In my mind these are pretty strong and valid "personal beliefs".

Now for the bad news. Even with these thoroughly-legal exemptions, I still found a paragraph in the regulations that seems to have the potential to supersede everything else. A paragraph called, "When exemption from immunization not recognized" (a bit of Tarzan-English I realize, but it's not my quote). What it basically says is that all of your "rights" as stated above can be taken away if, and I quote here:

"At any time there is, in the opinion of the state department of public health and environment or local department of health, danger of an epidemic from any of the communicable diseases for which an immunization is required pursuant to the rules and regulations promulgated pursuant to

section 25-4-904, no exemption or exception from immunization against such disease will be recognized. Quarantine by the state department of public health and environment or local department of health is hereby authorized as a legal alternative to immunization."

What? Did you know this stuff? The "quarantine" thing, and the ability for someone to overrule all your rights to exemptions? I didn't. Where, oh where are the conspiracy theorists on this one? In other words, all of your legal and civil rights, even your *religious convictions*, can go right down the drain if some random State or even local department of health Bozo (no offense to clowns) decides that there is a "danger of epidemic" for something you can get a vaccine for (and what *can't* you get a vaccine for these days) and thus can overrule you about your own health! Does this include the flu? Colds? SARS, bird flu, swine flu...excuse me – H1N1...(can't insult pigs), Billy Goat fever, Smelly Sneaker Syndrome or any other manufactured "scary disease du jour" that someone comes up with?

And if you still refuse the vaccine, it is then legal for them to "quarantine" (read *"imprison"*) you if they feel like it! Does this scare the dickens out of anyone but me? Maybe I watch too much futuristic Sci-Fi kind of stuff, but isn't this an awful lot of control of your own life to turn over to anyone? Am I the only person who saw the movie "V for Vendetta"? Doesn't it seem to anyone else that it feels like the pharmaceutical companies are coming up with diseases just so they can sell us yet another vaccine?

If this quarantine thing seems far-fetched to you, consider this: There is currently a system being put in place by State public health departments for use in every State (using federal funding) called Vaccination Registries. The purpose of this is to track every child born in order to monitor his or her vaccination status. Since this monitoring system would be in place in every State, there would be no way to get away from it. Even if you move, you'll be tracked from State to State by the linked systems. Wonderful, and how convenient.

Currently in place is the threat that without vaccinations your child might not be able to attend public school, but this new system will take it even farther. No shots? Okay. Then no school, no welfare, no food stamps, in fact no federal or State assistance whatsoever for the child or their whole family. One legislator from Oregon has even gone so far as to introduce a bill stating that unless parents can prove that their children have had all the government-imposed vaccines they can't file their children as dependents for their State income taxes! Where did this guy go to school? George Orwell U? Home of the Fightin' Big Brothers?

When U.S. authorities rounded up people during World War II just because they decided it was "safer" for the public, they called the facilities "internment camps", and this event is now considered a national disgrace. With one hand these government agencies give you three very sound reasons for exemptions, then with the other snatch them away simply because some person in a State or local department of health has decided to take away your personal, civil, moral, religious and legal rights, or because he or she just wants to. But don't worry, if they force poison into your body, or imprison you if you don't do what they want, it's for your own safety! You'll be *safer*. Whew! What a relief.

Ben Franklin has a quote about safety that I like. In 1759 he said, "Those who would give up essential liberty to purchase a little temporary safety deserve neither liberty nor safety." Right on Ben!

One last note on the "quarantine" issue. It brings to mind for me that these people must not really have much faith in these wonderful vaccines that are intended for our protection! If the vast majority of people are getting the vaccine, and ergo will not get the disease, then why are they worrying about someone who isn't vaccinated? Here, I'll be even simpler:

Person A: Has vaccine against Syndrome Blah Blah Blah.
Person B: On personal choice, refuses the vaccine.

That night, Syndrome BBB goes rampant in the county! Every single person who chose not to get vaccinated now has a raging case of it – forcing them to lie in bed and eat soup and grape juice and watch M*A*S*H reruns for days on end, and some already sick people could even die from it. So? If the vaccine actually works, then no one who got vaccinated will get sick, right? So why bother rounding up the sick "dummies" that chose against it and imprison them? Aren't they just getting what was coming to them? **If the vaccine indeed works, why worry about people who are sick transmitting the disease to those who were vaccinated? Aren't they "safe?" Isn't that why they got the damn vaccine in the first place?** *And what about the people who rather unfortunately develop the "accepted side effects" from the vaccine that may be as bad as, or worse than, the disease itself?*

After taking some time to recover after writing that last bit, I think the next thing to do is to just give you some basic info on what is in vaccines themselves. This is very valuable information for many reasons. One of them being that I have any number of clients who object to blood transfusions on a religious basis who were very shocked to find out that some of their vaccines contain all kinds of yummy tissue treats like human diploid cells from aborted fetal tissue, monkey fetal cells, mouse brains, albumin from human blood, and guinea pig embryo cells.

One woman client of mine who had received a Hepatitis A vaccine on the insistence of her doctor, about exploded over this revelation! I told her I was surprised that given her religious beliefs that she agreed to a vaccine that contained human diploid cells, to which she paled and answered, "What?" Her doctor knew she would not take transfusions because of deeply-held religious beliefs, but told her she needed to take a vaccine, which contained cells from aborted human fetuses! When confronted, he said he was worried about her health. She was worried about her *soul*. Which do you think is more important to *her*?

And what about all the vegans, yogis and other vegetarians who think "meat is murder" who have no idea what's in these vaccines? I have people who are so concerned over these kinds of issues that they open and dump out their supplement capsules so they won't get any gelatin that may be made using beef hooves. How do you think they would feel if they knew they were being injected with fetal bovine serum or aborted fetal monkey cells?

While researching for a list of the organic and inorganic ingredients in vaccines, I ran across some that just seemed too ridiculous and outrageous to be true. So I went to an official federal government website and got a copy of the "Vaccine Excipient & Media Summary" report. Imagine my shock when I saw row upon row of the very same "ridiculous" ingredients listed there too! Some of them have "explanations", but some of them... sorry, just can't figure them out. Why would you need "brilliant green" and "phenol red" dyes for color, and ingredients like aspartame and MSG? Aren't those all for appearance and taste? Did the formulator forget that these concoctions are for *injection*? If you thought eye of newt and wing of bat were darkly strange, take a close look at this report.

Mercury and aluminum and formaldehyde...oh my! Believe me, the more you research what vaccines contain, the less you'll want them injected into you or your family members. Just the sheer amount of lawsuits with plaintiffs numbering in the hundreds on each case should be enough to make you stop and think. Of course you won't see the name "mercury" on the list. It's called "thimerosal" and it's listed as a "preservative". Aluminum and aluminum adjuvants, which are now known to cause nerve cell death and therefore are commonly considered possible contributing factors to many neurological diseases (most notably Alzheimer's), can also be found in vaccines. Did someone forget that these are heavy metals? And *formaldehyde*? That's the main ingredient used for embalming people! Isn't it a bit precipitous to inject formaldehyde in a live person? (hmmm, "anti-aging" indeed!)

And then we come to the MMR – the Measles, Mumps and Rubella vaccine, which is one of the "Big Daddies" of the vaccines of concern. There are literally thousands of pending law suits just for this one vaccine and its suspected connection to autism. With at least one out of every 100 kids in the USA (depending on the study) now being diagnosed with autism, I think it deserves serious investigation. What is it about the MMR? The mercury? The varied types of live virus? The human diploid tissue cultures? Hard to say. It's such a lovely mix to be injecting into your sweet little 12 to 18 month old child who doesn't yet have the biological system in place to mount a proper immune response to the microbes. And since they can't do this, they instead form a tolerance to the very agent they are immunizing against, which opens them up to a world of chronic illness later in life. Between the MMR and the DPT these poor kids are "adversely reacting" at alarming rates.

Currently, and legally, one-year-olds are being vaccinated with ten different viral and bacterial agents at the same time. This is something I can totally assure you that the still-forming immune system is just not up to handling. And lest you forget – "adverse reactions". The minor ones like fever, headache, pain at the injection site, etc. are discussed to an extent, but the same "adverse" reports list paralysis, shock, brain damage and death. In other words, your child may develop seizures, autism or brain damage, and might die, but thank goodness he or she will have a far lesser chance of getting the measles!

And if vaccines are so good, then why does research from experts such as Dr. Russell Blaylock show that unvaccinated children are so healthy? Mothers of many unvaccinated children report that by pre-school or kindergarten, their children have never even had to see a doctor. I'm an adult example. I wasn't vaccinated and I rarely got even slightly sick. Vaccinated children on the other hand wind up seeing doctors frequently for all the telltale signs of shaken-up immune systems such as allergies, ear infections, asthma and eczema. I can't believe how many toddlers I see who have hideous eczema. I even saw one case where a little boy's eczema was so severe it was preventing him from walking!

The links between vaccines and neurological and other disease is huge, undeniable and mounting every day. Studies are being done from the U.S. to New Zealand to Russia and they all say the same things: Adverse reactions to vaccines are causing (among others) brain damage, seizures, autism, paralysis and death. Some research, including the amazing ground-breaking work being done by the aforementioned neurosurgeon Dr. Russell Blaylock among others, is even linking childhood vaccines to the current adult population explosions of chronic fatigue, neurological problems, and the immune system-related problems like rheumatoid arthritis, cancer, asthma, lupus and AIDS.

So where is the outcry? Where are the mobs of people and the media demanding that these things be taken off the market until more research can be done? They are either silent, or being silenced, or being denied. Vioxx® was implicated in the deaths of many thousands of people before it was finally pulled from the market. How many people have been damaged or killed by vaccines, which still remain "mandatory"? The Vaccine Adverse Event Reporting System revealed (and there are lots more findings that go unreported) that during a 20-month period, there were 54,000 injuries, hospitalizations or deaths as a result of vaccines. Where is the horror that people usually express when innocent children are being maimed, sickened and killed? Why are there actual laws being enacted to mandate that vaccines are given, instead of holding these drug companies accountable or demanding to know what's in the things?

Instead of horror we get the National Childhood Vaccine Injury Act. This piece of work was passed by Congress back in 1986 acknowledging "officially" that vaccines can cause injury and death, and was put in place – drum roll, please; *to protect both doctors and vaccine manufacturers from personal injury lawsuits!* This is the perfect scenario for vaccine manufacturers. Since the vaccines are mandated by the government, they can't be sued for the damage they cause. Protect Big Pharma and doctors. Just who's protecting our kids?

Since inception of this Act, despite having paid out well over a billion dollars in compensation to families, *three out of four applicants are turned away*, which begs the question: What kind of "proof" needs to be presented for them to pay out this billion dollars?

I work with one of the "turned away" ones; a girl (now 21) who was perfectly fine and healthy until receiving a round of her childhood vaccines. The same night following a vaccination, she started having seizures and has had them ever since. She is diagnosed with Lennox-Gastaut syndrome, a very severe form of epilepsy, and is completely confined to a wheelchair unable to move or speak since that day. Prior to having the vaccines she had never experienced seizures, but the doctors still deny that her neurological condition is in any way related to her vaccines. As I said before, what kind of "proof" is necessary? I think this needs to be taken into account in the already appalling statistics of what *is* reported as an adverse effect. And hey – at least she didn't get measles! Thank goodness for that! She could have been sick for days.

Although this damage seems most appalling when inflicted on little kids, there are far-reaching effects for adults as well. As it turns out, some of the very early polio vaccines were infected with Simian Virus 40, or SV40 as it is known, which has been shown to produce cancer in humans. At a National Institute of Health conference, several researchers showed evidence that they are culturing this very same SV40 from the brain, bone and lung tumors of both adults and children suffering from rare types of these cancers. It is also being speculated that it was the same monkey kidney cells used for this polio vaccine that were infected with Simian Immunodeficiency Virus (SIV) and that recombined with human genetic material to form Human Immunodeficiency Virus. Yes, HIV. The virus that causes AIDS, possibly brought to you by your friendly neighborhood vaccine. Many people diagnosed with HIV say that they have no idea how they contracted it. Doctors call this "denial", but it could be "vaccines".

Even the lowly Flu Shot, which people seem to line up like sheep for and has thus far not been very effective in preventing flu, has been linked to all kinds of neurological problems in adults, especially Alzheimer's and Guillain-Barre syndrome. Why? How about aluminum. Here people are avoiding fish and certain cookware to try to avoid mercury and aluminum poisoning, yet are lining up and paying to have those very same metals injected into their bodies in far more concentrated doses!

An interesting side note here regarding this last paragraph. To make sure I was spelling "Guillain-Barre" correctly, I looked it up in my "Dictionary of Medical Terms". In addition to describing it as "a form of peripheral polyneuritis marked by pain, weakness and sometimes paralysis of the limbs that may spread to the trunk of the body", it also said exactly this, and I quote, "The cause is unknown; it usually develops one to three weeks after a viral infection or immunization." Can you believe it? It actually says "unknown cause" then says it "usually" (*usually*, like commonly) develops after a viral infection or *immunization*! Isn't this kind of like saying, "The cause of the bruise was unknown, but it usually develops one to three hours after banging your shin on the coffee table?" These people get millions, sometimes billions of dollars to do research, and this is what they come up with?

While we're on aluminum, I have to tell you that this whole thing with this new HPV (Human Papilloma Virus) vaccine has got me really freaked out. I tried to do some research on it and couldn't find much, but what I found was a mess (another bad day for my staff I'm afraid). Apparently the NVIC was just as up in arms about this as I was, and I pulled this data from them. The test groups were small and the adverse effects were exceedingly common with about 90% of recipients reporting some adverse effects within 15 days. Yet the Governor of Texas decided to make it *mandatory* for all girls between nine and twelve years old in his State. I'm flabbergasted that a little-tested vaccine becomes mandatory on the chance that it *could* help in the prevention of HPV, which *might* cause cervical cancer, according to its own information provided in writing and on TV. What ever happened to choice?

The testing procedure alone on this vaccine is enough to arouse my suspicion. Usually in the oh-so-important placebo-controlled tests, the placebo used is an inert saline solution. For some reason in this case the FDA allowed Merck (the manufacturer) to use a placebo solution that contained potentially reactive aluminum. That means that nearly as many people reacted adversely to the placebo as to the drug (about 85% on the placebo).

Why do that? Well, it certainly makes the drug look safer and better! "We only saw a 5% increase in reaction over the placebo", certainly sounds better than "We had adverse reactions in 90% of recipients", doesn't it?

When most of us hear the word "placebo" we picture a harmless non-reactive compound of some sort (i.e. a sugar pill), right? Well they certainly hedged the bet on this one! There is 225 mcg of aluminum in the vaccine itself, and as of this writing, neither Merck nor the FDA would disclose how much aluminum was in the "placebo." They certainly changed the definition of the word "placebo" for their own purposes, didn't they? Kind of like saying that a soft drink won a taste test against Drano®.

Not only do I take issue with this vaccine, but also with the HPV itself. HPV (Human Papilloma Virus) is a sexually transmitted disease that can potentially be implicated as a cause of cervical cancer. If it was my nine-to-twelve-year-old daughter, I'd be pretty ticked off at the Texas Gov who assumed that my daughter was going to, at the age of nine, contract a sexually transmitted disease. And let's play "what if" for a moment. What if a girl had a dream to become a nun. Ergo, she is planning on never having sex in her entire life, and therefore would not be exposed to an STD. What right does the government have to force her to have a vaccine for something she thinks she'll never need? And on the other hand, let's say a girl is dreaming of being a mommy. She looks forward to one day getting married and having several kids. She gets the vaccine and it causes one of its listed known side effects – PID (Pelvic Inflammatory Disease), which has an unfortunate side effect of sterility. Sorry kid, no kids. Is this a vaccine or a form of forced sterilization?

As with all vaccines, there is frequent use of the words "may prevent" and "chance of", but, using HPV vaccine as an example, there is one thing that there is a 100% chance of – you will have HPV virus injected into your body. I thought the point was to avoid it! And then there is the "sexist" angle of this. Boys, although they can be carriers of HPV, are NOT being injected (yet). The apparent reasoning behind this that is since boys don't show symptoms of this virus, they don't need to be vaccinated. It seems to me that if they vaccinated boys, then they couldn't give it to girls, right? I mean who do you think the girls are getting this sexually transmitted disease from anyway if not boys? Keep in mind that I am against this thing for anyone – male or female, but what's the logic of just inflicting the girls with this?

It's amazing how many parents I know who would throw a fit if someone gave their child a Twinkie®, or let them eat something off the floor, but insist that they be injected with a noxious tonic of heavy metals, sugars, yeasts, colors and human and animal tissue cultures. Where is the reason in that? Avoid fish, but get vaccines? Huh? Yes, it is true that without the vaccines your child could get the flu, measles, mumps, chicken pox or even something serious like hepatitis or diphtheria, although they still could get the same things *with* the vaccine as well – *no vaccine promises to be 100% effective*. And by having them there is the chance that you or your child could have seizures, autism, brain damage, serious neurological damage, chronic lifelong illnesses, or even die. Which do you feel you need to be more afraid of? You choose.

Just like every encounter with a virus or bacteria, every encounter with a lab-altered virus or bacteria has an inherent ability to cause injury, illness or death. You could be exposed to all kinds of diseases over the course of your life, and then again you may not. By taking the vaccine you definitely will.

Please take the responsibility on yourself to find out what's in vaccines and what the associated risks are before you expose yourself to them. If you won't do it for yourself, then at least do it for your children. They trust you. Be worthy of that trust.

CHAPTER 12

The Popeye Protocol

"When diet is wrong, medicine is of no use. When diet is correct, medicine is of no need."
— Ancient Ayurvedic Proverb

"If there was a cure for Autism, everyone would know about it"
— Pretty much everyone

This chapter is only the tip of a very large iceberg. There is actually an entire forthcoming book I'm trying to finish up that will be solely based around the six years (thus far) of craziness that has ensued in my life resulting from this work. Something that I thought would be so easy to gain acceptance for and help with, has instead proved to be nearly impossible. Six years that (literally) very nearly drove me crazy because I just couldn't accept the level of resistance that I've experienced in getting the medical world to care about this. I lectured, I wrote, I gave interviews, I panhandled, we gave away our dietary recommendations to the world for free, and still...

Since making this discovery that confirms what vital impact diet has on the formation, reversal and prevention of Autism Spectrum Disorders as well as many other "mental" conditions in children and adults, I have received scientific awards, been lauded as a "Health Hero" (thank you Deborah Ray of the Alliance for Natural Health), and in 2009 was even Knighted for my work. What I *haven't* received, is much needed help on this.

The width and breadth of who knows about this work would astound you. I have met with extremely wealthy people who give millions to charitable organizations who told me that this "just wasn't up their alley". I've met with doctors who have either large segments on news networks or their own television shows who have seen proof of the success of my work and called it "interesting", nothing more. I've tried to show the same filmed evidence of the validity of the diet to the largest of the autism organizations to no avail. I've had large multi-national corporations including some of my product vendors promise to "give me any help I needed" who have never given me a dime or a hand. And as much as I hate to admit it, I've even had very influential people in the natural healing community who have shown just as much disregard for divergent thought as the allopathic community. Ouch...

As much as we hate to admit it folks, money talks. As disgusting as it may sound, we all know that to be a fact. The logical mind might attempt to dismiss any motivations for anyone to drag their feet so to speak in finding the real and effective answers for autism and related disorders, but after our six year journey, we have had to at least factor in and consider *all* the following. Just ask yourself:

Is it *possible* that many allopathic practitioners may be resistant to the notion that autism may be effectively addressed using short term, inexpensive and even home-implemented strategies? In example, seeing DAN (Defeat Autism Now) network practitioners can often cost families many thousands of dollars per month for indefinite years of care. What type of consideration goes into accepting that they should heavily diminish or lose that type of steady income? I'm just saying here...

Is it *possible* that those in the news station/network television industry have as a primary motivation the concern over helping to expose new and boat-rocking information that would risk or lose large chunks of their core Big Pharma, fast food, and breakfast cereal advertising sponsorship?

Is it *possible* that certain autism organizations might be blind-sided to finding answers for autism that primarily involve using better diet and other natural means as opposed to seemingly end-less research for more drugs and protracted therapy models, be-cause they could see losses of significant portions of their tens of millions in annual corporate and public donations as well as their jobs? *"Come on"* you might say, but it has been recently reported by the media that executives of certain not-for-profit autism ad-vocacy organizations are earning as much as high six figure an-nual salaries. Autism has become a tremendously large industry.

It is *more than possible*, that many of the "natural" information people just don't like the fact that my work wasn't their idea or discovery, although one prominent figure did tell me that he might consider helping if he could figure out "what was in it for him". My response was, "How about in helping to save a genera-tion or more of children?" Insufficient answer I guess.

As awful as all that is to believe, at least I sort of get it. Money is everything to many, and autism has become very big and po-tentially perpetual business. The only people who really feel for us are the parents, and even that support is inconsistent in the following circumstances:

1. The parents whose child has successfully been through our protocol, losing most or all of their ASD symptoms along the way, who then refuse to talk about it. I can't tell you how many people will not even mention to their child's school or doctor that they have even been on the protocol or write a testimonial for us! SO MANY just want to pretend that the whole thing never even happened. The amount of shame, guilt and negative stigma that is attached to these syndromes is unbelievable. You'd think we were working with STD's, not ASD's!

2. The parents who refuse to believe the up-close-and-per-sonal-in-their-face *proof* that this works because they don't seem to want to change their own lifestyle habits. This, my friends, BLEW MY MIND! As an example; the people who watch as

their next door neighbor or sister or friend heals their child of their ASD symptoms with this dietary protocol and then still deny that it did anything because they don't want to change their own ways. Instead of changing some dietary and lifestyle habits (i.e. *cooking* instead of pouring something out of a box or can) they would appear to prefer to leave themselves, or their own children, autistic. Are cereals and breads *really* that important?

This is (again literally) the stuff of nightmares for me.

At first I felt that I had discovered this *missing link* by chance, but then I remembered that I don't believe in coincidence. I wasn't looking for it, so it found me instead. The result of this research has been the most amazing and rewarding thing I have ever done or may ever do, and my life, as well as the countless lives of clients who have decided to give the program a solid try, have been improved because of it. I strongly encourage you to investigate this. Go ahead – it's been totally free to access since Thanksgiving of 2009.

So, here's the story behind the Popeye Protocol

In June of 2005, a tired and frustrated Mom brought her three-year-old son into my office. He had been diagnosed as "autistic" in October of 2004, and though she had no expectation that anything could be done to help his autism, he had some digestive issues she wanted to try to address in the hopes that there might be some positive modification in the wild nature of his behavior if he started feeling better. He was the first autistic child I had ever seen as a client.

The diagnosis of autism is a permanent brand not only on a child but on the whole family. This little guy had started out life well, and at the age of one he seemed to be more advanced than slow. He walked at an early age and had been adding words to his vocabulary on a nearly daily basis. This all halted abruptly one day after he was taken in for some routine childhood vaccinations. The day after he had his DPT, MMR and HIB vaccines, he spiked a fever and was exhibiting flu-like symptoms. The doctors assured his Mother that this was a "normal" reaction to the vaccines, but it was anything but normal from there on. He never spoke another word after the vaccines, and a few months later the diagnosis was in – Autism. The relation to the vaccines was determined to be merely "coincidental".

Since I just brought up the subject of vaccines, which seems to rightly be such a hot-button topic these days, this is as good a place as any to make clear my general feelings about them. As a Traditional Naturopath I obviously am not wild about injecting any unnatural substances into the human body (I do not take vaccines myself, nor does my family) and would encourage anyone out there to do a very thorough investigation on vaccines before making your own educated choice. If you decide to do this, an excellent place to start is at The National Vaccine Information Center at www.nvic.org.

However having said that, I am far from pointing an exclusive finger of blame at vaccines as the primary precursor and sole culprit for promoting these conditions along the Autistic Spectrum. Although I do feel that they can be a contributing factor, and perhaps in some cases the major factor, my experience leaves me unconvinced that they are the only factor in the recent rises in incidence. Also, as a Naturopath, I am far more interested and involved in finding solutions to given symptoms and conditions than in pinpointing their exact diagnosis or reasons for occurring. That's what this Protocol is all about: Regardless of how the condition originated, this has been a way to start reversing and repairing damage.

While I have had any number of behaviorally-challenged children in my office, this boy really was a wild child. Despite the fact that his Mother firmly attempted to keep control of him, he was extreme. He tore around the office touching and smelling everything like a little animal, and would suddenly scream for no apparent reason and claw at his Mother. He was terrified of me, which made my assessment of him even more of a challenge. His Mother, in his defense, explained that he was terrified of all female doctors because of multiple incidents with a woman doctor who was very rough with him and had even performed a minor surgical procedure on him (snipping off a piece of foreskin) without the benefit of anesthesia. The doctor told the horrified Mom when this happened that "Autistic kids don't feel very much." Do you think she wondered why the kid was screaming his brains out if it didn't hurt? It was no wonder the kid was scared of me or any doctor!

This story however, is what first struck me odd about his "autism". Autistic children in general are nearly completely indifferent to their surroundings, including a marked indifference to people. Why then would he only react with fear to *female* doctors, and not to males? Or how would he even recognize that a person was a doctor in the first place? I don't wear a white coat or any other identifying "doctor things", and my office just looks like any other office and even lacks that distinctive "doctor's office smell" that so intimidates most of us.

So, if he was exhibiting the usual detachment from others that most autistic children do, then why or how would he even make these distinctions? This made me look for more examples along the same vein. Although there were plenty of consistencies with classic autistic exhibited in his behavior (i.e. his outbursts and tantrums, a complete lack of intelligible or even unintelligible speech, and most noticeably his overactive senses), his unusual male/female/doctor distinction was enough to make me look for more inconsistencies.

I found plenty. As I said, autistic kids are usually quite indifferent to their surroundings; the core basis of autism is that they live in their own world. Instead, this kid was investigating everything he could get his hands on: Smelling, feeling, and even tasting, once taking a bite out of a large plant in my office. He played for a long period of time with a toy that often confuses adults, his motor skills were excellent, and he watched me like a cat, often making long-term eye contact with me. He showed plenty of diverse emotions by both cuddling with his Mother and then showing clearly that he was terrified of me. *None of this fit with the accepted pattern of autism.*

And even though extremely heightened sensitivity to touch, light, smell and noise is consistent with autism, it struck me that even though the physical touch from his Mother seemed to hurt him, *he kept returning to her when feeling the most frightened*. It was as though even if it hurt, the comfort was worth the pain. Again, not the uncaring and "in-their-own-world" behavior of autism. Already I was on my toes with this one.

As I've eluded to before, in my office we perform what we call our "BioBaseLine® Assessment" on all new clients. This includes using a piece of noninvasive, bio-resonant/bio-feedback computer interfaced technology that is a highly advanced system that can greatly help me with assessments. In a nutshell, it doesn't test for specific levels of toxins, insufficiencies or excesses in the body like blood test standards, but rather looks at the body's *stress reactions* to any given exposures.

An example of this concept I often give to people is demonstrated by sensitivities to peanuts. Some people can eat them by the handful, while others can go into anaphylactic shock if they eat something that once sat *next* to a peanut. The *amount* therefore is not the sole important factor, but the *reaction* is always the key. The conclusions that can be drawn using this system are understandably different from what standard tests might reveal, and since I don't diagnose, the information it supplies me with is many times invaluable.

So, with this little boy during the course of this assessment process, one word kept popping up repeatedly on the computer screen – manganese. I didn't give it much thought the first few times it showed up, since mineral, enzyme and other nutrient names show up often. After repeating itself several times, I wrote it down as a note on his test sheet.

A little info about manganese is warranted here. Manganese (Mn) is one of those nutrients you don't have to give a lot of thought to, as many foods contain manganese and the body usually regulates it on its own. Generally there will only be a mere 12-20 mg. stored in the body at any one time. It is a naturally occurring mineral that is found in many types of rocks. Referred to as the "brain mineral" it is important to the utilization of all the mental capacities and functions, as well as in the formation of tendons, ligaments and in maintaining the structural integrity of the lining of various organs. Obviously the "brain mineral" idea caught my attention. However the recorded signs of manganese deficiency, such as carpal tunnel, deafness, tendon weakness and retarded growth rate did not seem to apply in this particular case.

After the family left my office, the word "manganese" continued to intrigue me. Enough so that after office hours I pulled out the boy's chart and went over it again and again. Something was bothering me, but I just couldn't figure out what. I looked for the small things on his chart that sometimes get overlooked in the hectic and limited confines of an original appointment, especially with a kid charging around eating my plants.

When I asked if he had any allergies, his Mother said no, but noted that "He throws up if he eats either soy or blueberries." Looking up soy and blueberries in a nutritional handbook, I found they are both "excellent sources" of manganese. However, my further investigation revealed that manganese *excess* is known to inhibit iron absorption, and the boy had many low iron symptoms. It started to make some sense. This wasn't likely to be a case of manganese deficiency, but it may be a case of manganese excess!

Looking for problems associated with manganese excess in standard nutritional handbooks yielded next to nothing, so I turned to the Internet. Among others I found articles from the Weston A. Price Foundation and David Goodman, PhD, both addressing a condition called "Manganese Madness". According to numerous studies, the primary site of collection for manganese toxicity, *regardless of the source of exposure*, is the basal ganglia; a mass of nervous tissue nestled within the cerebral hemispheres of the brain. This attributed cause and effect was first proposed by an English physician who in 1837 noted that some of the workers in a local manganese mine appeared "lethargic and their faces unexpressive". Since neurological textbooks identify manganese as a neurotoxic metal, the disease of "Manganism" was coined by the turn of the 20th century.

According to what I could initially locate on "Manganism", this disease that struck manganese miners exposed to toxic dust appeared to cause symptoms of "emotional liability, irrationality, hallucinations and impulsivity." Chronic exposure led to "muscular weakness, ataxia, tremor, immobile facial expressions, and extreme speech disturbances." These symptoms, which sounded a lot like Parkinson's in adults, seemed to me to be suspiciously similar to autism in a child. Further reading revealed that other very common symptoms of manganese excess can be speech difficulties and extreme reactions to sensory input: Light, touch, smell and sound. Now *that* all seemed to describe my young client perfectly.

The more research I dug up, the more fascinating and clear it became to me. Could this be a source of this boy's symptoms? All the reports described it perfectly! Something that might be encountered by an adult as "emotional liability" and "problems with speech" could very well be perceived as insurmountable to a child barely more than a year old. And my little client's most prominent symptom, the overwhelming nature of his sensory input, was described in each and every report. Limiting and annoying to an adult, I could completely see how terrifying it might be to such a young child.

The one thing that my research was revealing absolutely nothing about was how to counter such an excess. Could there be a way to defeat the manganese overload and thereby halt these negative symptoms? My hunting through medical research papers revealed little or no information or help, so I fell back on the number one tool available to a Naturopath – my own intuition. Because excess manganese can be indicative of low iron and/or result in inhibited iron bioavailability, it made perfect sense to me that additional dietary iron might help to displace and start balancing the excess manganese.

At this point I decided to phone the boy's Mom and desperately hoped that she wasn't going to think I was crazy for suggesting what I was about to ask of her. I described the course of thought I'd followed on this and the results of the research that I'd completed so far. Then I told her my wild idea that just maybe if we loaded up her son with dietary iron (I didn't want to use supplements at this point) it might possibly overwhelm the manganese and restore balance, thereby reducing his sensory overload symptoms. Things got pretty quiet there for a moment while she considered what I was saying, and I held my breath hoping she'd agree to try it.

Her first question back to me was simply concerning how she would be able to get all the iron into him. Exhaling in relief, I started explaining my plan. This boy heavily preferred fruits and vegetables over any meats in his diet, and I had already done a quick check to prepare a short list of some vegetables and fruits highest in iron that included such items as spinach, apricots, cherries and almond milk. I also reminded her to load his diet with good fats (especially olive and flaxseed oils), try to get him to eat more quality meats, and told her I was sending her some Spirulina in order to try to speed up the iron-loading process.

She expressed some doubt as to whether he would eat these new foods ("Don't all kids hate spinach?"), but assured me she'd do her best. I suggested that she let him play with his food, eat with his hands, whatever it took, and asked her to please keep me up to date on any reactions or progress.

Ten days after his original appointment, only nine days on the high-iron protocol, his Mother called as promised to give me her first progress report. First of all to her surprise, he was loving the diet. She described him as "eating like a horse" and happily scarfing down all the iron-rich foods I had recommended. Once a picky eater, he now looked forward to mealtimes. As I had suggested, she was letting him "play with his food", eat with his hands, whatever, as long as he ate it, and in particular he was consuming raw spinach with gusto. She told me that he was carrying it around and eating it right out of the bag with both hands "like potato chips". I asked if anything in his behavior had changed, and she began giving me her positive report. Already he was slightly less sensitive to light and touch, and had stopped smelling everything "like a puppy dog".

In our entire conversation, there was an undertone of... something. She sounded excited, which I could understand, but there was something else. So I asked, "Is there something else? Any other changes?" This was the question she was waiting for to spring her news on me: "Just one – he's started to talk again!"

I was thunderstruck. Talk? In nine days? At first I didn't say anything and she started to laugh. At my urging she went enthusiastically on and on, describing "the big moment". Her son had been eating a raw spinach salad rather energetically and with great enjoyment, and held his plate out for more. She asked him, "Did you eat all your salad?" and without hesitation and in a completely clear voice he said "I eat it all." Shocked, she responded, "What did you say?" He pushed his plate out and asked "More?" She buried him in spinach! *These represented his first spoken words in nearly two years.*

When I next saw him in my office, it had now been 28 days after his original appointment. This was a different child. The first thing I noticed was that he shyly said, "Hi Dr. Young" (with a little coaching from Mom) when I walked in, but the changes ran much deeper than that. While still in the waiting room he engaged with other people, saying hello or handing them magazines. His Mother reported that he was starting to mimic others (very comically mimicking his Father) and was making the connections to words at a very fast pace. For example, he pointed at a lamp, and his Mother told him the word for it. He said "Lamp", then switched it on and said, "Light. A lamp makes light." Most notably, his "wild" behavior had diminished almost as soon as he started talking. Once he could express himself he lost the manic energy that kept him running in circles, clawing at people or himself and screaming. His sensitivity to input was still a little high, but as his Mother put it, "No longer inappropriate."

Two months after his original appointment, they came in with some truly wonderful news. After some tests, the boy had been "reclassified" by his doctor as "not autistic" and he was starting pre-school in the coming semester. They had found him a therapist to help him catch up on his speech and he was progressing very quickly. Less than three months into my work with him, I discharged him from having to see me regularly.

At the time I originally wrote this chapter (2008), this boy was in a regular pre-school doing very well, although they were considering home-schooling for him because of his recently discovered high IQ. His sense of humor, energy, focus and appetite had remained high. His Mom continued to call in once in a while to let me know how well he was doing physically and how well his sense of humor was continuing to develop. The last I saw of him, he was very friendly, social and no longer afraid of me. I guess he finally figured out I wasn't going to hurt him.

Unfortunately, this was one of those "break my heart" cases I spoke of. An interesting side note on this case was the very divergent reactions of those on both sides of the "natural medicine" issue in the family. The Mom became a true believer and the last I spoke to her she was actually considering schooling to become a Naturopath. However, Dad and most notably, Dad's Mother, felt that it was just a "coincidence" that the boy recovered at the same time that we began the dietary protocol. It's amazing what lengths people will go to in order to stay comfortably within their existing paradigm. By the way, you'll find the written testimonial from his Mother among those on our foundation website www. noharmfoundation.org.

After the spectacular results with this case, I dug into this idea with a vengeance. Every moment I wasn't seeing a client and much of my after work time became consumed by investigating this subject; both my poor dogs and my staff bravely bore the brunt. My next major area of exploration was; where did such a little kid get so much manganese? He obviously wasn't a miner, so that was out! Further research started turning up some other possibilities. For example, soy-based baby formulas (which my little client had been fed) can contain 200 times the amount of manganese naturally-contained in human breast milk. No wonder their little bodies might go into overload.

Two tragic accidents in London hospitals should have alerted more in the medical world to the potential dangers of soy formulas overloading manganese into the brains of infants. Two babies suffering from liver damage were fed nutrient solutions containing small amounts of manganese through their intravenous feeding tubes. Even though the manganese concentrations were no greater than that in soy baby formulas *and were therefore considered safe by government standards*, the actions were attributed to causing brain damage after feeding periods of only a few months.

John Donaldson, a toxicologist and speaker at a UC Irvine conference, described how manganese overload steps up the brain's electrical charge, increases its virulence ten-fold and attacks vulnerable dopaminergic neurons. Francis Crinella, Clinical Professor of Pediatrics also at UC Irvine, had gone so far as to propose that manganese overload might prove to be an explanation and contributing factor behind the epidemic of adolescent violence currently sweeping the country.

Once I had more of this knowledge under my belt, I started to be on the lookout for symptoms and for the easily identifiable issues that always were present during my consultations. To my surprise, I started finding them not only in kids, but in adults as well. The first adult who seemed to have the same markers was a very nice 47-year-old guy with some rather odd symptoms. He came to me looking for help with persistent "borderline high" blood pressure, frequent insomnia, and a head tic he had recently developed.

After noticing some paranoid behavior from him, my questions revealed that he was experiencing "more paranoia than I want", and even stranger was doing a great deal of involuntary scenario-building in his head. As an example of this, he had seen what he thought might have been his wife's car parked in front of a real estate office in town (note: you can't swing a cat in our town without knocking over a real estate agent!) and in moments he had an entire story unfolding in his mind wherein his wife was leaving him for a real estate agent, the guy was going to "have him killed", his kids were going to wind up working in a factory, on and on!

As you can imagine, this was pretty scary to him. Strangely enough, he displayed all the exact same issues that had been present in the little kids. I figured, why not? So I explained the concept of why this might happen, and gave him the very same food and supplement protocol that I was using with kids, but obviously with a few dosage adjustments due to the fact he was a full grown man. He was intrigued and said he'd try it.

Within a few months, he managed to kick not only his input overload issues (like the scenario building and bad dreams) but also his physical issues. As it turned out the blood pressure, insomnia and tics may have primarily resulted from his bottled up anxiety over his involuntary and unexplainable behavior. He reported feeling "totally cool now" and to his relief had given up, as he put it, "building evil castles in the air." As experience has proven, this type of paranoia is present in a vast majority of affected people, both kids and adults. I've dubbed it "Worst Case Scenario" building, and it can get pretty extreme.

My experience with the adults was opening my eyes to all kinds of new vistas. With kids I had already seen fantastic changes with everything from autism, ADD, ADHD and good ol' undiagnosable rotten behavior, to anxiety, nightmares, anger issues and insomnia. In adults I was now seeing the exact same identifiable issues with people who had received diagnoses of schizophrenia, bipolar disorder, Parkinson's and Alzheimer's as well as the more nebulous, but common, "I think I'm losing my mind" complaint. And the uncanny part was I was observing the almost identical nature of what I had come to think of as my "markers" in every affected person regardless of his or her age.

The main difference was that what I had dubbed the "Popeye Protocol" seemed to work slightly quicker on the kids than the adults. I think this is easily explained in three ways: (1) Kids generally have no mental attachment to illness and therefore merely let go of symptoms without questioning *why* they feel better, as most of us over-thinking adults do, (2) the older the person or child is, the more ingrained patterns and habits become and the harder they are to break, and (3) since they are not the ones in charge of the selection and preparation of foods, their diet, being *the key* to the Popeye Protocol, can be more closely regulated to produce faster results. Unlike adults, three and four-year olds rarely grab fast food on their way home from work!

Again, the question of the hour remained; where was all this manganese coming from? None of these adults were currently taking any soy baby formulas, and not a single one was a miner, so...? Since I'm a Naturopath and not doing what is considered to be empirical evidence-based work (it's not like people are throwing buckets of money at me to research this), I've been kind of on my own here. As one of my happy "autism Moms" put it in a particularly succinct and amusing way at the end of two months of having her child on the protocol, "I only have one question – why aren't you on Oprah?" Well, for one big thing, I'm not an *MD* like Dr. Oz and others.

Research money is rare for natural practitioners like me, as is recognition by scientific or media sources, so I had to continue looking for these symptoms where I found them among my already very full schedule of people instead of having the luxury of seeking out just the ones who had a good chance of exhibiting this syndrome. I continued to be shocked at the variety and number of such people I encountered.

So although I didn't know for certain at the time, I began to develop the belief that in most cases the excess of manganese may be more attributed to the lack of bioavailable iron in someone's diet than to high consumption of or other exposure to manganese. I also became more and more suspicious that often the culprit might be a low-iron diet *coupled with excessive vitamin consumption*, as many commercial vitamin products contain ludicrously high amounts of manganese, which is generally considered to be only a "trace" mineral in requirement.

It's worth reiterating here that there's a potential with many supplement enthusiasts is to take up to an entire line of products, such as those produced by many network marketing/home business marketing companies. Understand here that I am *not* knocking network marketing companies – I'm just cautioning people who combine an insane amount of products together! As I've said before, many times less is more when it comes to vitamins and supplements. People forget that many nutritional products are formulated by their manufacturers to be "stand alone" supplements, and therefore typically contain the full DV of minerals such as manganese. Take a whole bunch of these products together, and you can take in a whole lot of manganese (as well as other potential overloads).

One of the more common emotional markers I have noticed in adults is that some of them obsessively and compulsively control their diets and are inordinately paranoid about their health.

One young woman who had become obsessively worried about food additives was pretty much living on soy products and handfuls of multivitamins. No mystery as to the source of her particular overload.

It would not be for a few years down the line that we discovered what I now consider to be the primary and underestimated culprit in the formation of this imbalance that I have now named the "Menefe Syndrome", which is dietary consumption of phytic acid salts known as "phytates". Phytates are anti-nutrients found to various degrees in grains, legumes, seeds and nuts that tightly bind to many minerals and make them unavailable for absorption and use in the body. Analytical chemists actually use purified phytates in experiments where it is necessary to isolate and quantify the amounts of elements like calcium, magnesium, zinc or iron present in a sample because the phytate binds to these ions tighter than just about any other molecules. Unfortunately the very same thing happens when you consume phytate in foods, and this can have a very harmful effect on many bodily aspects such as proper growth, bone health or iron status.

So consider that anything made from grains, like breads and cereals, can be loaded with high amounts of phytate. In other words, nearly everything that most Americans are used to eating for breakfast is causing their iron and many other necessary minerals to chelate out without being utilized, which among a myriad of consequences, leaves receptor sites in the brain open for business for available manganese. There is well documented research and evidence that in the case of insufficient iron and surplus manganese, brain transport mechanisms will resort to substituting manganese in brain receptor sites that are intended to function with iron (visit www.noharmfoundation.org for plentiful research). No wonder we're drowning in an Autism tsunami!

So am I saying that my dietary therapy will work with *all* autism, all ADD/ADHD, all chronic depression, all Parkinson's cases? Of course not. However, I am saying that it has proven to me to be extremely effective when a component of a person's problem may be excess manganese. I will also say that the food protocol, used all by itself without supplementation, has produced everything from mixed positive results to full reversals and rediagnosis. In many of the kids and most of the adults there were also other health conditions present that needed to be addressed; most notably leaky gut syndrome (one of the Syndrome markers), which also negatively affects your iron absorption and utilization.

After hearing one of my lectures, many people have gone home and tried the food protocol with their kids without employing any other means of immune system or digestive tract support. The results have ranged from slight to significant enough for them to bring the kids in to see me from all across the country. The food is the key, but sometimes it needs some added personalization and specialized help.

One thing that all these disparate syndromes in both kids and adults seem to have in common is that they all generally result in substantial financial burden and hardship. Part of the beauty of this protocol is that most of the components are *just foods*, and therefore completely affordable as you have to buy food anyway.

So let me pose this question: Why not just check for excess manganese in these cases? Before putting people on lifelong protocols of very serious and expensive drugs with very serious side effects, why not check for this imbalance *first*? Or even lacking hard biomarker evidence of that, why not just get a person on this high iron protocol and see if there is any positive result? The usual response time for the first significant changes to be noticed is averaging between 9 and 14 *days*, and no one in this world is going to be damaged by a few weeks on a very healthy, high-iron and phytate-free diet.

In fact, why bother with an invasive and/or expensive test that will only show amounts and not *sensitivity* (like the peanut thing again) when the protocol itself couldn't cause any harm? I've seen tests all over the board that showed "high" manganese levels when a person had no symptoms, and "normal" manganese in a heavily affected person! There just isn't any rhyme or reason when individual sensitivities are in the mix.

Conversely, the same can *not* be said about the usual drugs that people are put on for these conditions. The side effects for the drugs suggested for these specific conditions are enough to make anyone sick, and the number of prescriptions written every year for them climbs ever higher. The common ADHD drugs (that are given to little, *little* kids, for heaven's sake) are mostly amphetamines and more recently, seizure medications that carry severe warnings including insomnia, nervousness, rapid heartbeat, depression, and added in the case of Adderall®, addiction, seizures, stroke and *sudden death!* Want proof? Look it up! Not to mention that Ritalin®, Focalin® and Adderall® all carry a listed side effect of "toxic psychosis indistinguishable from schizophrenia" and the growing concern about the suicide rate among these kids. You really want to put *that* in your four year old?

And yet despite the added risks, despite the fact that Adderall® is being referred to as "college crack", the number of prescriptions written continues to go up and up! According to IMS Health (who conducts health-care-market research) sales of Adderall® went up 3100% between 2002 and 2005 alone!

And think about this: After you've had little Janey or Johnny on uppers since age five or six, do you think he or she is going to be able to "Say No To Drugs" in their teens and beyond? Fat chance after years and years on legal meth supplied by the friendly neighborhood pushers – in this case, none other than dear old well-intentioned Mom, Dad and the family doctor! And keep in mind, we are talking about a *legion of kids*. Although more boys than girls are on these kinds of drugs, girls are gaining *fast*, as evidenced by a 2010 Medco Report that showed an increase of 40% between 2001 and 2010 for girls. That's a lot of "addicts in training", if you ask me.

Strangely enough, this report also showed an increase in the use of these same ADHD meds by women between age 20 and 44 of 264% between 2001 and 2010. Is this a case of "mother's little helper" or are they simply continuing an addiction that started when they were still in pigtails?

And the drugs for adult conditions aren't any better, though at least adults make the choice to take them instead of having them forced upon them by schools, doctors and parents. Most Parkinson's drugs carry warnings of hallucinations, difficulty breathing, confusion and jerky movements. Is it just me, or does that sound a lot *like* Parkinson's? Alzheimer's drugs all offer the not-so-comforting prospect of providing "<u>some</u> *temporary* relief in <u>some</u> cases"– hardly a ringing endorsement, along with some very serious side effects like breathing problems, hallucinations, irregular heartbeat and seizures. And the most commonly prescribed anti-depressants all come with their usual side effects of gastric disturbances, sleep disorders, weight gain, sexual dysfunction and suicidal ideation. I don't know about you, but any one of those would be enough to depress me! As with many prescription drugs it seems that the side effects on these are as bad as or worse than the conditions and diseases themselves. Especially if we can discover that what this person really needed – *was spinach!*

So, is anyone still asking why this was originally called the "Popeye Protocol?" Just in case, I'll illuminate. It actually started out as a joke in my office, then just stuck. Two of the main components of this dietary protocol, to whit; dietary iron and fatty acids, are exactly what Popeye knew was so good for him: Spinach, and olive oil (or Oyl in his case). Turns out he was right.

The dietary portion of the protocol is now referred to as the Spectrum Balance® Protocol (SBP) Diet. If you would like your own current copy, it is available for free download at <u>www.no-harmfoundation.org</u>. Read it for yourself, and make your own call. Apparently no one else is going to do it for you.

CHAPTER 13

How the Popeye Protocol Became The Spectrum Balance® Protocol

Sorry folks. That's a whole other book…

Coming soon…

CHAPTER 14

Quack!

"The superior doctor prevents sickness; the mediocre doctor attends to impending sickness; the inferior doctor treats actual sickness."
— Chinese Proverb

The derogatory appellation "Quack", once my nemesis, has its basis in the Dutch language. The marketplace hawkers of "snake oil" and other "cures" were so loud that they sounded like quacking ducks to shoppers, hence the term. However, I have another take on it. How about:

Qualified
Under-rated
And
Caring
Keepers of Life

My subtitle of this book, "Confessions of a Naturopath" was my little joke. Usually a book that starts with "Confessions of..." has a naughty or shameful cast to it, and as so many people consider the art and practice of natural medicine to be somewhat shady, I thought it was appropriate. Hopefully this book will go a long way toward enhancing public information and clearing the name of competent practitioners of the natural arts.

So now that you've read my book and have a better idea of what we do, do yourself a favor: Go get your phone book and look in the Yellow Pages under "Naturopaths".

Go ahead, it's OK. We're almost done and I'll wait here.

See? There we are...

Maybe Naturopaths will always be considered quacks, but I sure hope not. Either way it doesn't matter much to me any longer. Speaking for myself and many other dedicated healers, we will keep doing exactly what we do no matter what labels society and government hang on us, or how much grief they try to hand us. I never have and never will care about empirical evidence. I care about *results*, and I've had a great many of them; and I'm fully devoted to continuing to have them, to give them. I've seen people with prognoses of a few weeks or a few months live to complain a year later that they still (still!!) have to struggle to finish a half hour on the Stairmaster! I've seen "autistic" and "behaviorally challenged" kids rapidly talk, read and be loving, intelligent and sharing children. I've seen people on walkers, crutches or in wheelchairs get back to their lives and into the gym. And I've seen those with "incurable" diseases walk away whole and happy to live to cheat on their diets. And the babies, well, I've have many "impossible" conceptions with healthy babies as the result under my belt. Because of the laws I couldn't help once their Moms got pregnant, but I did help them get there! My picture appears in several of my clients' family photo albums. It doesn't get any better than that.

So here's a message to all you Naturopaths and other healers out there – those of you who wake up every day knowing that you're in for a fight, but get up and do it anyway because you love it and because you believe in what we do, hear this: Stay strong, stay with it, and be proud of yourself. This is important work that we do.

I am a Naturopath; a healer by any name you might call me, and I'm proud of it. I am happy with what I've done and what I will do in the future. And if Naturopaths are quacks, then I'm definitely a great big duck. QUACK QUACK! Take that...

Be well...

Acknowledgments

As with any big project, there were a lot of people involved in making it happen. I'd particularly like to mention my editor for the original writing, Lisa Schofield, who not only did a great job in smoothing out my sometimes choppy thoughts, but who was also the first "outsider" to really love this book.

Neither this book nor any of my work could happen without my team and family of the Assertive Wellness Center. My Mom came out of retirement (yet again) and answered the phones before I could even afford to pay her, then used her own special gifts to create an environment where people felt welcome and cared for. Judy Crews handles the craziness of both me and my front desk and continues to help further our internal research. My brother Doug used his creativity and gifted expertise to build a business from my dream. And his lovely wife Lori stepped in where we most need her with her expertise and exhaustive research on nutrition. Truly, this is the Dream Team!

On a personal note, I really want to thank my parents, Larry and Doris Young. You taught me how to create and trust my ideals, when to stand and fight and when to beat a tactical retreat, and most importantly, how to love myself and others. Without your love, support and sacrifice there would be no book, and no doctor.

More grateful nods go to my other support teams. To Dr. Mark Smith at the University of Natural Medicine for his invaluable and kind help, and for repeating to others, over and over "It's her head". To Bill Cunningham for his constant willingness to help. To Christy Whitlock, one of our first online support group moderators extraordinaire who has been invaluable in learning and answering many questions for parents and giving my work one thing I never could; the oh-so-important

"Mommy-cred". To Linda Kane who always reminds me why I do what I do and has showed so many the way to recovery; she's an angel. To Glen White for thinking I'm invincible. To Kingsley Gallup who taught me how to be "right sized", and to Rachael and David from Landmark Education for helping me to have what it takes to be unreasonable enough to write a book like this.

The most special of my thank you's must go to Doug Young, Chairman of the NoHarm Foundation. Aforementioned fabulous brother, best friend, rock star of business managers, and my un-failing (and unflailing) Rock of Gibraltar no matter how stormy the seas. No one could wish for a better brother, researcher or friend. He has been there for me every step of the way since my first steps, and I will always be deeply grateful.

And of course, to my amazing clients who have traveled to see me from all across the country and around the world. You trusted me not only with your health, but with the lives of your precious loved ones. Your health was my goal, your trust has been my reward. I am honored, and I thank you all with all my heart. This book has been a blessing to write as it reminded me of so many people and times I don't often think about, and it is about you, and for you.

There is a Cherokee saying that being loved deeply gives you strength, and that loving deeply gives you courage. I have been blessed with both. Thank you all.

Made in the USA
San Bernardino, CA
25 February 2015